Practical
Equine
Dermatology

Practical Equine Dermatology

Second Edition

Janet D. Littlewood
Veterinary Dermatology Referrals
Cambridge, UK

David H. Lloyd
The Royal Veterinary College
Hatfield, UK

J. Mark Craig
Re-Fur-All Referrals
Newbury, UK

WILEY Blackwell

This second edition first published 2022
© 2022 John Wiley & Sons Ltd

Edition History
Blackwell Science Ltd. (1e, 2003)

Registered Offices
John Wiley & Sons, Inc., 111 River Street, Hoboken, NJ 07030, USA
John Wiley & Sons Ltd, The Atrium, Southern Gate, Chichester, West Sussex, PO19 8SQ, UK

Editorial Office
9600 Garsington Road, Oxford, OX4 2DQ, UK

For details of our global editorial offices, customer services, and more information about Wiley products visit us at www.wiley.com.

Wiley also publishes its books in a variety of electronic formats and by print-on-demand. Some content that appears in standard print versions of this book may not be available in other formats.

Library of Congress Cataloging-in-Publication Data Applied for

[PB: ISBN: 9781119765486]

Cover Design: Wiley
Cover Image: © Janet D. Littlewood, Kieran O'Brien

Set in 10/13pt Palatino by Straive, Pondicherry, India

Printed in Singapore
M113701_131221

Contents

Preface to the second edition

This second edition of *Practical Equine Dermatology* updates the text of the first edition and provides information on a number of new diseases. Although much of the information has not changed, it has provided the opportunity to increase greatly the number of illustrations whilst focusing the text more closely on diseases of the skin. Thus, diseases of the foot and associated structures have now been incorporated within the other problem-orientated chapters, and conditions that are primarily orthopaedic have been omitted. In addition, suggested references and further reading are presented at the end of each chapter in order to make them more readily accessible to the reader, rather than as a single block at the end of the book.

As before, the aim has been to provide a concise, problem-orientated text facilitating a well-organised diagnostic approach together with a basic presentation of equine dermatology in a practical format illustrated with pictures of the principal conditions, particularly those in which visual information is an important part of diagnosis. All of the conditions likely to be encountered in the UK are included, and information on some rarer conditions, such as those that may occur in imported horses, is also provided. However, detailed information on rare and complex diseases is not included as it is anticipated that such conditions will require referral to a specialist in equine dermatology.

Indications for treatment are given within the text. These are generally based on UK practice and on products available within the UK. Where unlicensed preparations are mentioned, readers should understand that these should be used only when licensed products are not available and that efficacy and safety of unlicensed products and 'off-label' use cannot be guaranteed. Issues relating to drug use in horses are considered in the final chapter on Therapy in Equine Dermatology.

This edition has been revised principally by Janet Littlewood and David Lloyd, with assistance by Mark Craig. Sadly, 'Tommy' Lovell Thomsett, who was a pioneer of equine dermatology in the UK, has passed away. However, his knowledge and wisdom remain as an important component of the book.

The authors hope that this text will not only provide practical help on the everyday problems of skin disease in equine practice but that it will also stimulate a deeper interest in equine dermatology.

Janet D. Littlewood
David H. Lloyd
J. Mark Craig
March 2021

Acknowledgements

The authors would like to acknowledge colleagues at Rossdales Equine Hospital and Practices for their generosity in contributing images and for support and advice during the preparation and updating of this edition of the book. They relied on the Royal Veterinary College Dermatology Group slide collection and also wish to acknowledge in particular contributions from the late Dr Keith Barnett, Dr Malcolm Brearley, Dr Harriet Brooks, Mr Andrew Browning, Dr Greg Burton, Dr Alistair Cox, Ms. K. Clarke, Dr Emily Floyd, Dr Marcus Head, Dr Sandeep Johnson, Dr Ewan Macauley, Professor Celia Marr, Mrs Jacqueline Mortimer, Dr Kieran O'Brien, Dr Richard Payne, Dr Rob Pilsworth, Dr Oliver Pynn, Dr Stephen Shaw, and Dr Liz Stevens.

Disclaimer

While every care has been taken by the authors and publisher to ensure that the drug uses, dosages and information in this book are accurate, errors may occur and readers should refer to the manufacturer or approved labelling information for additional information.

Readers should also note that this text includes information on drugs that are not licensed for use in horses. Readers should therefore check manufacturers' product information before using such drugs.

The diagnostic approach

A structured approach is essential. Vital information is obtained during the history-taking process and sufficient time must be allowed for this. Accurate information on husbandry is particularly important. Clinical examination must include systemic and skin components. The process is illustrated with flow diagrams (Figures 1.1 and 1.2).

TAKING THE HISTORY

The approach (Figure 1.1) is similar to that adopted in other species. Points to include are:

- Breed, age, sex, origin:
  - Consider these aspects carefully; in many conditions, these simple data will have an important impact on your diagnostic considerations.
- History of skin problems in related animals.
- Type of husbandry and use:
  - Length of time owned.
  - Use – competitions, general riding, breeding, racing.
  - Feeding regimen.
  - Periods spent in stable or at pasture.
  - Type of stable and bedding – stable hygiene, contamination.
  - Conditions in paddocks – mature meadow pasture or new grass ley, proximity of water, trees.
  - Seasonal changes in management.
  - Routine health care procedures – vaccination, deworming.

Practical Equine Dermatology, Second Edition. Janet D. Littlewood, David H. Lloyd and J. Mark Craig.
© 2022 John Wiley & Sons Ltd. Published 2022 by John Wiley & Sons Ltd.

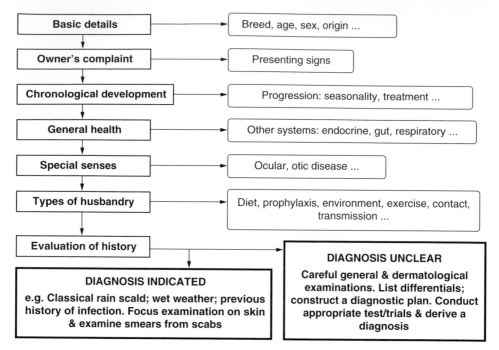

Figure 1.1 Taking the history. Components and the sequence of the history taking process. Analysis of the history should enable the clinician to construct an initial list of differential diagnoses that may help to focus the clinical examination along particular diagnostic lines. It may enable the diagnostic process to be abbreviated where a likely diagnosis is indicated, or it may point towards the need for a more detailed approach.

- Grooming procedures – sharing of grooming kit, tack, grooms.
- Equipment used in contact with horse – boots, bandages, saddle cloths, rugs.
- Contact with other horses, other species – opportunities for disease transmission.
- History of the current problem.
  - First signs, progression, response to treatment and management changes.
  - Seasonal effects.
  - Previous episodes of disease.
  - Results of any diagnostic tests.
  - Current or recent therapy – includes questions about use of over-the-counter and non-veterinary products.
  - Evidence of transmission – lesions in other horses, other species, humans.
- General health – concurrent or previous conditions.

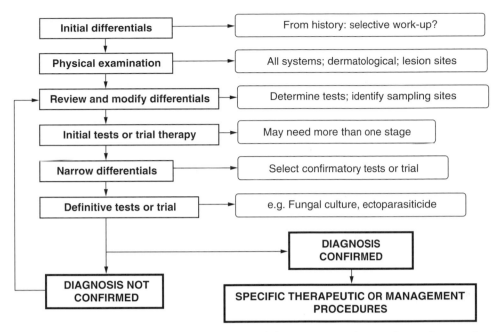

Figure 1.2 Clinical examination and diagnostic procedures. A thorough general and dermatological examination should be carried out unless the history points clearly towards a diagnosis. Examination coupled with history enable a list of differential diagnoses to be drawn up, formulation of a diagnostic plan and the selection of appropriate tests and sites to be sampled, and/or therapeutic trials.

CLINICAL EXAMINATION

A full clinical examination to assess both the general health status and the skin is necessary in most cases. Ensure that the animal is adequately restrained and that you have sufficient light. Work systematically down each body region, beginning at the head and ending at the tail and perineal region. Be sure to include all aspects of the feet including the coronary band and the frog. The skin may need to be cleaned to observe some lesions. In some instances, sedation may be necessary.

A record of the distribution and severity of primary and secondary lesions should be kept. Forms including a horse outline make this much easier (Figure 1.3).

It may be helpful to visit and examine the paddocks and exercise areas used.

EQUINE DERMATOLOGY EXAMINATION FORM

Horse:...   Date:.........................

Owner:...

Distribution
of lesions

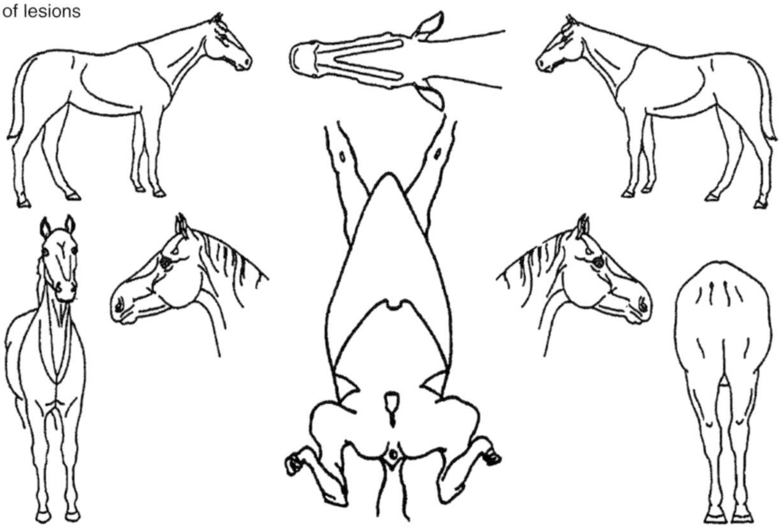

Owner complaint:

Description of lesions:

Differential diagnoses:

Diagnostic tests:

Figure 1.3   Example of an examination form for recording distribution and nature of lesions in equine dermatology cases.

DIAGNOSTIC TESTS

The history and clinical examination should enable you to formulate a list of differential diagnoses. It may help to create a problem list, identifying the relevant historical features and predominant clinical signs, categorising them as contagious or non-contagious, and allocating the disease within the following groups, which form the basis for the problem-orientated approach in this book:

- Pruritic
- Crusting and scaling

- Ulcerative and erosive
- Nodular or swollen
- Alopecia/hair coat changes
- Pigmentary disorders

A diagnostic plan can then be constructed, diagnostic procedures selected, and samples collected. Sample collection may include the following techniques.

Hair plucks

Useful to determine whether the lesions of alopecia or hypotrichosis are due to self-inflicted damage (fractured hair shafts, split ends) indicating that the condition is pruritic, or due to abnormal hair growth (absence of anagen roots, abnormal catagen roots), and to examine for dermatophytes and for parasite eggs.

- Choose fresh, unmedicated lesions.
- For suspected dermatophytosis, where cultures are required, first lightly clean the areas to be sampled with 70% alcohol (to reduce contaminant organisms).
- Tissue or epilation forceps can be used to grasp gently and pull out hairs from the periphery of the lesion.
- Samples for microscopy can be placed on adhesive tape wrapped around a microscope slide and mounted in a drop of liquid paraffin just prior to examination.
- Samples for fungal culture submission should be held in paper or sterile, non-airtight containers to prevent a humid environment that might support the growth of saprophytic organisms.

Crusts

Useful for cytological examination looking for bacterial organisms (particularly *Dermatophilus*) and for submission for fungal and bacterial culture.

- Choose a fresh, unmedicated lesion.
- Impression smears of the underside of freshly removed crusts, stained with a rapid Romanowsky-type stain (e.g. Diff-Quik, Hemacolor, Rapi-Diff, Speedy-Diff) or Gram's stain, can provide a quick method of diagnosis for dermatophilosis.

- Crusts can be collected and held in paper envelopes or sterile containers for transport to the laboratory.
- Dried crusts can be emulsified in a drop of sterile saline on a slide, warmed to allow rehydration of material, prior to air-drying and fixing (heat fixation for Gram's stain, methanol/ethanol fixation for rapid-differentiating Romanowsky-type stains) for cytological examination and identification of bacterial and fungal organisms.

Coat brushings

These allow for examination for surface-living external parasites and dermatophytes where the lesions are diffuse or extensive. Scrapings are better for deeper resident mite infestations.

- Use a sterile scalp brush or new toothbrush to brush firmly over the lesions (Mackenzie brush technique; Figures 1.4a and b). Place the brush in a paper envelope to protect it prior to submission for dermatophyte culture.
- A scalp brush or wooden tongue depressor can be used to collect debris directly into a sterile Petri dish for external parasites. Material should be examined promptly as chorioptic mange mites are highly motile and easily lost from sample containers.

(a)   (b)

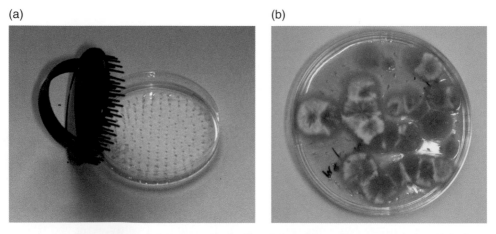

Figure 1.4   (a) A coarse-toothed brush (e.g. 90 mm Denman scalp brush) facilitates sampling of large areas of skin and coat. The collected hair can be removed and examined, or the teeth may be embedded in a fungal culture medium as illustrated. (b) Here *Microsporum canis* has been isolated using this technique.

Skin scrapings

Skin scrapings can be performed for detection of external parasitic diseases such as chorioptic mange, larval stages of harvest mites, demodicosis (rare), or for dermatophyte culture and cytology.

- If necessary, remove hair over areas to be sampled by careful clipping.
- Use a wooden tongue depressor for superficial sampling or a large, curved scalpel blade if deeper samples are required, with the sharp edge blunted to reduce the risk of injuring the horse or operator.
- Moisten the sample site or the collection tool with liquid paraffin (more useful for examination for mites), water or normal saline (for dermatophytes).
- Gently scrape crusts, scales, and associated hair so that the material accumulates on the blade or tongue depressor. Transfer onto a microscope slide with more liquid paraffin, or with potassium hydroxide solution if collected in aqueous medium, which allows clearing of debris and easier identification of pathogens.
- Deeper scrapings are needed for suspected demodicosis, deep enough to cause capillary ooze.
- Sample several sites, collect plenty of material, and divide amongst several slides to make thin suspensions, which are quicker and easier to examine efficiently.

Surface adhesive tape samples

An alternative method for obtaining surface material, including *Oxyuris equi* eggs, surface-living ectoparasites, hair fragments, exfoliated cellular material, and surface microorganisms for direct microscopical examination or after staining; it is less traumatic and avoids the risk of injury associated with skin scrapes. This technique is particularly useful for identification of chorioptic mange mites which are highly motile, but also allows detection of other pathogens including dermatophytes and yeasts.

- A piece of clear adhesive tape (e.g. 3M Scotch Crystal, Sellotape Clear) is applied to the lesional area 3–4 times (Figure 1.5).
- Tape is applied (sticky side down) to a microscope slide over a drop of liquid paraffin for direct examination or over a drop of blue dye from a rapid Romanowsky-type stain kit.
- Excessive mounting medium or stain is removed by wiping with soft paper towel prior to microscopical examination.

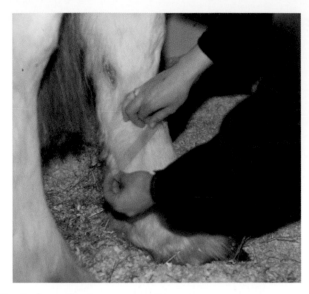

Figure 1.5   Surface adhesive tape sampling.

Direct smears

From fresh, exudative, crusted, excoriated, or pustular lesions, a direct impression smear can be made for cytological examination and for microorganisms.

- Press a glass slide against the concave undersurface of a removed exudative crust, or against the surface of a freshly exposed lesion.
- For an intact pustule, gently break the overlying skin with a 25 g needle and press a clean glass slide to the ruptured lesion, or purulent material may be collected in the needle bevel and then transferred to the glass slide.
- For lesions at sites where it is difficult to apply a slide directly, material can be collected with a dry swab and then rolled onto a glass slide.
- Air-dry the slide and store in a slide box prior to heatfixing (for Gram staining) or immersion in methanol (for Romanowsky-type staining).

Wet crust preparations

For older, crusted lesions this technique enables microscopical examination of dried exudate.

- Representative sample of crust is placed on a glass slide with a few drops of normal saline.
- Material is finely chopped and macerated with a scalpel blade.

- Slide is left in a warm place for 20–30 min to allow rehydration of cellular material.
- Any large clumps of debris are gently removed prior to thorough drying and heat fixing of the remaining suspension prior to staining with a rapid Romanowsky-type stain kit.

Swabs

May be useful for bacteriology and fungal culture and collecting material for cytological examination.

- If the sample is to be processed within 30 min of collection, a dry, sterile swab can be used for bacterial and fungal culture, and smears. Otherwise, place swabs into suitable transport media (e.g. Amies charcoal medium, or Copan ESwabs).
- Samples collected from the skin surface may not be representative of the causative agent, so collect pus from an intact pustule or the underside of a freshly removed scab, or submit biopsy material for culture. Useful cultures may sometimes be obtained from a dry crust by rehydrating with sterile normal saline prior to processing.

Needle aspirates

This technique is used for sampling nodules, masses, and enlarged superficial lymph nodes.

- A 20–22 g needle can be used, with or without a 5 ml syringe. The area to be aspirated should be carefully cleaned and disinfected.
- The needle is inserted into the nodule (Figure 1.6), mass, or lymph node and used to probe the tissue in several places, initially without aspirating, and subsequently whilst gently aspirating.
- The needle is withdrawn from the tissue and detached from the syringe, which is then filled with a small amount of air, reattached to the needle, and the sample expressed directly onto a clean slide for cytology or onto a swab for culture. A second slide is placed over the sample to spread the material. The slides are then separated gently to avoid damaging cells and air-dried prior to staining for microscopical examination.

Biopsy samples

Skin biopsies may be collected for a variety of reasons, including histopathology, fungal or bacterial culture, viral identification with electron microscopy, and immunohistochemistry. If in doubt, consult a pathologist as to the best way to process and transport the biopsy to the laboratory.

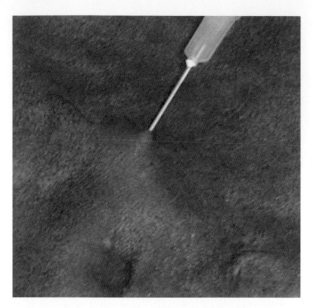

Figure 1.6   Fine needle aspiration of a nodular lesion. Source: Courtesy of Liz Steeves.

There are three common ways to take biopsy samples: by excision, biopsy punch (Figure 1.7), or shave biopsy (see Chapter 3). The most common is the punch biopsy technique described below.

- Sedation is generally necessary, followed by local analgesia. For the distal limbs, a nerve block (low or high four-point or abaxial sesamoid, depending on the area involved) may be performed or local infiltration below the sample site or as a ring block around the lesion. For facial and difficult to access sites, such as inguinal and perineal lesions, general anaesthesia may be required.
- Areas that include primary lesions should be selected where possible and sites not marred by medication. Take multiple samples unless only one lesion type and stage is present.
- Because sample orientation during histopathological processing cannot be predicted, ensure that the whole punch sample includes tissue of interest. If normal skin is to be included for comparison, this should be taken as a separate sample in an appropriately labelled pot. Where you wish to investigate the transition between lesional and healthy skin, take an elliptical excision sample with the long axis going from normal to abnormal.
- The selected sites may be marked using a coloured marker. Try to avoid areas overlying superficial ligaments, blood vessels, nerves, or superficial synovial structures associated with tendons and joints.

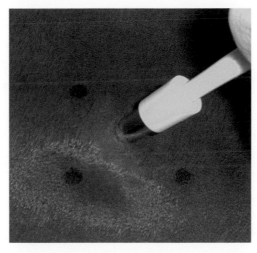

Figure 1.7   The punch biopsy procedure enables rapid sampling and is suitable for most equine lesions. Source: Courtesy of Harriet Brooks.

- *It is important not to prepare the site surgically before sampling, since this removes surface material which may be of great diagnostic value.*
- The selected site may be anaesthetised by injecting approximately 1–2 ml of mepivacaine or lignocaine hydrochloride without adrenaline into the subcutaneous tissue below the lesions.
- Wait for 2–3 min and test for sensation at the site with a needle.
- Use a 6–9 mm biopsy punch; generally, the larger the size of the punch is better. Ensure the cutting edge is sharp.
- Apply the punch with rotating movements in one direction to limit artefacts until through the skin, then withdraw. The sample may be attached to underlying structures by a thin attachment. Grasp the sample gently with small haemostat forceps or a hypodermic needle at the subcutaneous portion, lift from the surrounding tissue, and cut free using sharp scissors.
- Place the sample in the correct transport medium. For normal histopathology, 10% neutral buffered formalin is used. Keep samples for culture moist by wrapping in a sterile gauze swab soaked with sterile normal saline and consult the microbiology laboratory about the appropriate medium for submission.
- Clean around biopsy sites with diluted 2% chlorhexidine or povidone-iodine solution and suture using a single interrupted suture of 2–0 monofilament nylon. For sites where it might be difficult to remove sutures at a later date, an absorbable suture may be more appropriate.

- Topical antibiotic powder or spray may be used; bandages or adhesive dressings may be needed at some sites.
- Submit samples in appropriately labelled pots together with a fully completed submission form, including pertinent clinical history, in order to get the best value from your histopathologist and microbiologist.

Other samples

Collection and examination and/or analysis of forage and bedding may also be valuable.

Diagnostic investigations specific to individual diseases will be covered in the relevant chapters.

REFERENCES AND FURTHER READING

Cowell, R. and Tyler, R. (2001) *Diagnostic Cytology and Hematology of the Horse (2nd edition).* St Louis, Mosby Inc.

Sloet, M.M. and Grinwis, G.C.M. (2018) Clinical pathology in equine dermatology. *Equine Veterinary Education*, 30: 377–385.

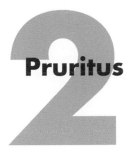

Pruritus

Pruritus is one of the commonest presenting signs in equine skin disease. It is manifested in many ways, which may be observed by the owner and deduced by the veterinary surgeon on examination of the affected animal. Such signs may include:

- Irritable demeanour.
- Restlessness.
- Kicking and stamping.
- Rubbing against objects.
- Biting the skin.
- Attempting to scratch with hind limbs.
- Hair loss, thinning, broken hair.
- Excoriation, exudation, crusting.
- Bruising, swelling, haematoma.
- Skin thickening, scaling.

The severity of pruritus may be difficult to gauge from the history. Use of a pruritus visual analogue scale (PVAS) may be helpful to document severity and monitor response to treatment (Figure 2.1).

Practical Equine Dermatology, Second Edition. Janet D. Littlewood, David H. Lloyd and J. Mark Craig.
© 2022 John Wiley & Sons Ltd. Published 2022 by John Wiley & Sons Ltd.

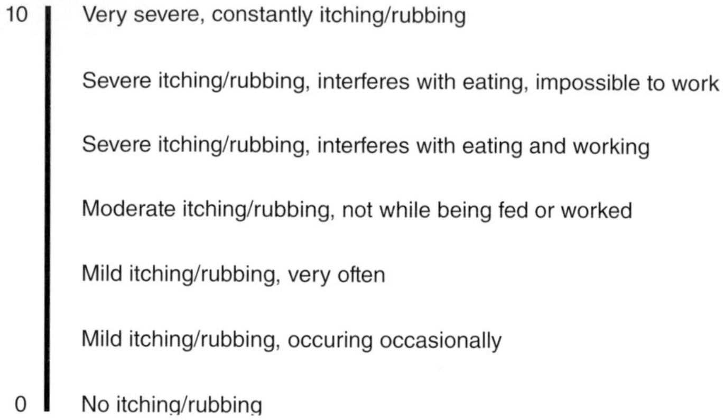

10 | Very severe, constantly itching/rubbing

Severe itching/rubbing, interferes with eating, impossible to work

Severe itching/rubbing, interferes with eating and working

Moderate itching/rubbing, not while being fed or worked

Mild itching/rubbing, very often

Mild itching/rubbing, occuring occasionally

0 | No itching/rubbing

Figure 2.1   Visual analogue scale for owner assessment of pruritus in their horse.

CONTAGIOUS CONDITIONS

ECTOPARASITIC INFESTATIONS

Louse infestation (Pediculosis)

Clinical features
- Mild to severe pruritus, patchy alopecia, excoriation, exudation, in-contact animals affected; ill temper, loss of condition, and, in severe infestation with sucking lice, anaemia.

Bovicola (Damalinia, Werneckiella) equi
- Biting/chewing louse: small (c. 1.5 mm long) with a rounded head, many lice usually present; affects the dorso-lateral trunk and neck, especially under the mane and on the head (Figures 2.2a and b), and the tail base. More prevalent in the winter months.

Haematopinus asini
- Sucking louse: large (c. 3 mm long), more easily seen, generally fewer lice; usually affects the base of the mane, tail, and fetlocks. Populations can be high with extensive infestations in long winter coats (Figure 2.3).

Diagnosis
- Signs, history (underlying problem causing debility?).
- Find lice and nits, identify microscopically.

Treatment and control
- Topical insecticides containing cypermethrin (5% concentrate in Deosect 5% w/v/Concentrate for Cutaneous Spray Solution, Zoetis UK; 2.5% in Barricade 'S' Dip and Spray, Zoetis UK), permethrin

(a)

(b)

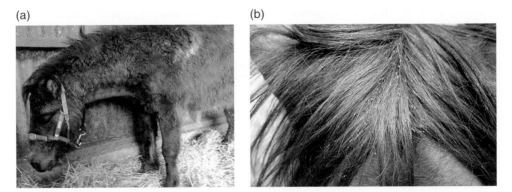

Figure 2.2 (a) Alopecia of ventral neck and poor hair coat in a pony with pediculosis. (b) Nits (louse egg cases) attached to the hairs of the forelock. Source: Courtesy of Kieran O'Brien.

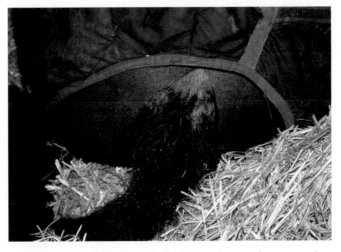

Figure 2.3 Alopecia and excoriation of tail base due to infestation with sucking lice *Haematopinus asini.*

(Coopers Fly Repellent Plus, MSD Animal Health; 4% w/v in Switch Lotion, VetPlus), or pyrethrins (Dermoline Insecticidal Shampoo, Battle, Hayward & Bower); at least two applications at 7–14-day intervals; pruritus controlled in <36 h, transient urticaria has been reported.

- 1% selenium sulphide shampoo shown to be effective for chewing lice, whole body shampooing repeated on three occasions at 10-day intervals, with contact time of 5–10 min before thorough rinsing; veterinary product Seleen shampoo is no longer available, human equivalent is Selsun Blue maximum strength, Chattem; (note that Selsun shampoo, Delpharm Bladel B.V., contains 2.5% selenium sulphide and might be irritant).

- Ivermectin oral paste (Noromectin, Norbrook; Eraquell, Virbac; Vectin, MSD Animal Health; Eqvalan, Boehringer Animal Health; Animec, Chanelle Pharma; Bimectin, Bimeda) 200–300 µg/kg, repeated after 14 days and 28 days for sucking lice.
- Pyrethroid powder (Barrier Louse Powder, Barrier Animal Healthcare): apply to whole body and work in with soft brush, repeat after 7 days.
- Fipronil 0.25% spray (Frontline Spray, Boehringer Ingelheim Animal Health) has been shown to be effective (off-label use) with elimination of all adult and immature forms reported after a single application.
- Treat in-contact animals, rugs, tack, and grooming kits; products containing cypermethrin suitable for use in agricultural environments are available.

Mite infestation

Chorioptic mange

Clinical features
- Infestation with *Chorioptes bovis* affects predominantly the distal limbs, but may spread to other regions. The hind legs are more often involved, and cob and heavy breeds are especially susceptible.
- Condition is clinically apparent particularly during colder times of year.
- Affected animals usually show signs of pruritus with stamping, and rubbing or biting at the affected areas, although some animals may show minimal pruritus.
- Lesions (Figure 2.4) include scaling and crust formation in the pastern, fetlock, and cannon regions.
- Exudative, proliferative dermatitis with secondary bacterial infection may develop in severe cases.
- One of the differentials for 'greasy heel' syndrome.

Diagnosis
- History and clinical signs.
- Demonstrate the mite in adhesive tape strips or superficial scrapings from fresh lesions (Figure 2.5) or at the edges of more chronically affected skin.

Treatment
- No licensed products for this disease in the horse.
- Topical treatments are best applied after clipping and cleansing to remove crusts; the following have been reported to be effective:
  - 1% selenium sulphide shampoo repeated three times at 5-day intervals, allowing a skin contact time of 10 min prior to thorough

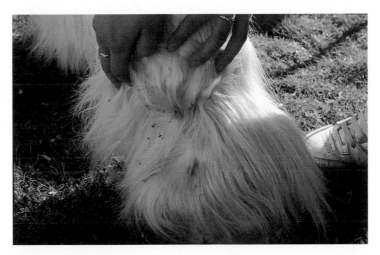

Figure 2.4 Haemorrhagic crusts and exudation affecting the pastern region of a Shire horse with chorioptic mange.

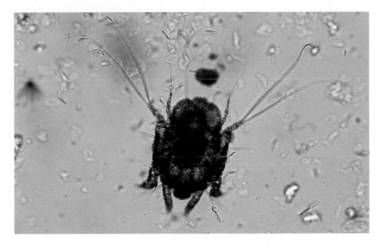

Figure 2.5 Adult female *Chorioptes bovis* in liquid paraffin (x125).

rinsing (Seleen shampoo is no longer available; human equivalent Selsun Blue maximum strength, Chattem; note that Selsun shampoo, Delpharm Bladel B.V., contains 2.5% selenium sulphide and might be irritant).
- Fipronil 0.25% spray (Frontline Spray, Boehringer Ingelheim Animal Health); apply sufficient to dampen skin and haircoat, repeat after 4 weeks.
- Sulphurated lime solution (Lime Sulphur Dip, Easi-Vet; Lime Sulfur Dip, Vetoquinol USA) applied as a 1 in 40 dilution of concentrate on four occasions at weekly intervals.

- Systemic treatments with published evidence of resolution of pruritus and >95% reduction in mite numbers include:
  - Doramectin (Dectomax 10 mg/ml solution for injection, Elanco UK AH) 0.3 mg/kg given by subcutaneous injections, two doses at 14-day intervals.
  - Ivermectin oral paste (Noromectin, Norbrook; Eraquell, Virbac; Vectin, MSD Animal Health; Eqvalan, Boehringer Animal Health; Animec, Chanelle Pharma; Bimetin, Bimeda) 200–300 µg/kg, repeated after 14 days.
- Other off-label treatments with anecdotal support include:
  - Ivermectin 0.1% solution in propylene glycol (5 ml of ivermectin 1% injectable solution in 50 ml propylene glycol) applied to each leg as a sponge-on after prior clipping and washing with medicated shampoo, repeated after 4 weeks.
  - Application of a small animal flea/tick collar impregnated with synthetic permethrin (e.g. Scalibor Protectorband, MSD Animal Health; Seresto Collar, Bayer Animal Health) to each limb; in case of contact reaction one limb only should be treated initially, and only collars with a locking buckle to prevent over-tightening and an elasticated section to prevent 'snagging' should be used.
- Treat in-contact animals and dispose of bedding to prevent reinfestation.

Sarcoptic and psoroptic mange

- Rare in Western Europe, but may occur in imported horses.
- A few cases of sarcoptic mange have been reported in equids in the UK and Sweden in recent years, with a history of contact with infested foxes. (Figure 2.6).
- *Sarcoptes scabiei* causes intense pruritus with papules, crusts, alopecia, excoriation, and lichenification, beginning on the head and neck and extending caudally. Infestation with the fox-adapted species appears to show lower risk of contagion than classical disease; successful treatment reported with doramectin injections; sulphurated lime solution is also likely to be effective, with repeated applications.
- *Psoroptes equi* causes severe pruritus, crusting, and alopecia, especially of the head (ears), mane, and tail. Rapid transmission occurs.

Psoroptes cuniculi infestation

- Can be found in horses' ears and may cause no problems or lead to head shaking and ear rubbing. Affected animals may have a lop-eared appearance.

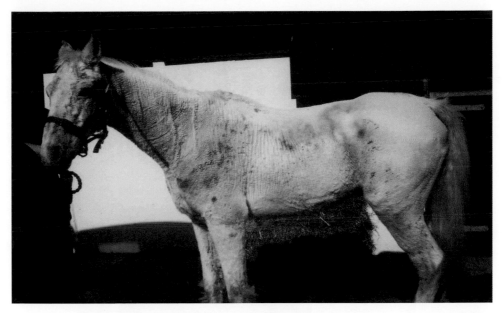

Figure 2.6 Pony showing extensive alopecia affecting head, neck, trunk, and hind-quarters with excoriations, erythema, crusting, and thickening of the skin with rugal folds due to sarcoptic mange. Source: Littlewood (2011), figure 1, p. 25. Reproduced with permission of Equine Veterinary Education.

Diagnosis
- Signs and history indicate an ear problem.
- Otoscopic examination of the equine ear is difficult, requires sedation and use of a flexible endoscope; mites may be seen as white moving dots.
- Confirmation of diagnosis by microscopical examination of debris from ears.

Treatment
- Clean debris and wax from ears.
- No licensed products available; oil-based ear drops for small animals likely to be effective (Canaural, Dechra Pharmaceuticals; Surolan Ear Drops, Elanco UK AH) or systemic endectocide such as doramectin injection (Dectomax 10 mg/ml solution, Elanco UK AH).

Free-living mite infestations

Trombiculidiasis (*Neotrombicula autumnalis* (harvest mites, chiggers, red bugs) infestation)

- Larval form is parasitic.
- Free-living adults found particularly in chalk grassland, but also in scrubland and wooded areas.

Clinical features

- Larvae usually acquired from infested pasture in late summer or autumn.
- Several animals in a group may be affected, with variable, sometimes severe, pruritus, indicated by stamping and rubbing.
- Signs include papules, wheals, and alopecia that may affect limbs, head, and the ventral abdomen (Figure 2.7).
- Larvae may be visible as orange-red dots (<0.5 mm) on affected skin. Larvae detach after engorgement, although pruritus may persist for longer.

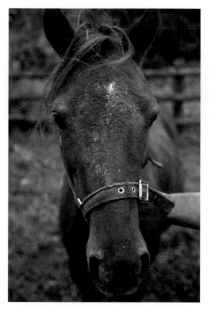

Figure 2.7   Patchy alopecia of face due to trombiculidiasis.

Diagnosis

- History, signs, demonstration of the six-legged larvae in surface adhesive tape samples or skin scrapings (Figure 2.8); sample other animals in same group, even if not particularly pruritic.

Treatment

- Larvae detach after feeding, but therapy is usually warranted. A single treatment with a topical antiparasitic preparation, e.g. fipronil 0.25% spray (Frontline Spray, Boehringer Ingelheim Animal Health), cypermethrin (5% concentrate in Deosect 5% Concentrate for Cutaneous Spray, Zoetis UK; 2.5% in Barricade 'S' Dip and Spray, Zoetis), permethrin

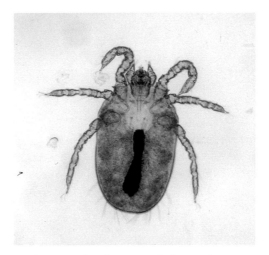

Figure 2.8 Larva of *Neotrombicula autumnalis* from a skin scraping.

(Cooper's Fly Repellent Plus, MSD Animal Health), or pyrethrins (Dermoline Insecticidal Shampoo, Battles) should be sufficient for current infestation, but repeat infestation possible; some residual preventative effect with two-weekly application of fipronil spray.
• If possible, areas infested with these mites should be avoided in the late summer and autumn.

Poultry red mite (*Dermanyssus gallinae*) infestation

Clinical features
• The red mite of poultry lives in the environment and buildings where poultry are kept or have access and emerge at night to take a blood meal; mites are not normally found on affected horses during the day.
• Pruritus occurs where mites bite, often affecting the head and limbs, and sometimes also the trunk (Figure 2.9).

Diagnosis
• Signs together with a history of contact with poultry housing are usually highly indicative.
• Mites are just visible with the naked eye; examine surface adhesive tape samples or coat brushings and scrapings taken at night.

Treatment
• As for *Neotrombicula autumnalis* infestation.
• Avoid areas close to poultry accommodation; horses may need to be moved away if the mite infestation cannot be eliminated.

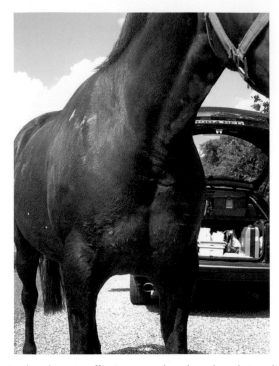

Figure 2.9 Patchy alopecia affecting ventral neck and trunk in a horse housed in building previously used for poultry. Source: Courtesy of Marcus Head.

Forage mite infestations

These free-living mites, e.g. *Acarus* or *Pyemotes* spp, may be present in hay, other forage, and bedding and thrive in warm, humid conditions.

Clinical features
- Can cause papular and crusty lesions, which may be pruritic, in areas of skin in contact with contaminated material, such as feet, muzzle, head and neck (hay in nets), trunk.
- Hypersensitivity component may be involved.

Diagnosis
- Differentiate from other papular and crusting conditions affecting feet and muzzle.
- Demonstrate mites (0.3–0.6 mm long) in adhesive tape samples, skin scrapings, and samples of forage and bedding.

Treatment
- Removal of contaminated material leads to recovery in a few days.
- Symptomatic anti-pruritic treatment may be necessary in some animals.

HELMINTH INFESTATIONS
Oxyuriasis

Clinical features
- Female *Oxyuris equi* worms emerge from the rectum and lay cream-coloured eggs on the perineum causing pruritus.
- The horse rubs its tail (rat tail) and becomes restless or ill-tempered.
- Infestation occurs especially in stabled horses where rapid transmission of the eggs can occur; eggs are sensitive to desiccation.

Diagnosis
- Signs are usually highly suggestive.
- Demonstrate presence of typical operculate eggs by microscopical examination of adhesive tape sample taken from perineum.
- Differentials: *Culicoides* hypersensitivity, pediculosis, atopic dermatitis.

Treatment
- Clean perineal region once or twice daily to remove eggs and break life-cycle, apply petroleum jelly to discourage egg-laying, and prevent eggs from sticking.
- Improve stable hygiene.
- Ivermectin paste (Noromectin, Norbrook; Eraquell, Virbac; Vectin, MSD Animal Health; Eqvalan, Boehringer Animal Health; Animec, Chanelle Pharma; Bimetin, Bimeda) 200–300 µg/kg by mouth or moxidectin gel (Equest, Zoetis UK) 400 µg/kg by mouth. Monitor efficacy of treatment by faecal egg counts and repeated tape strips 14 days later, routine faecal egg counts every 8–12 weeks as per current guidelines.
- Persistent *Oxyuris equi* infestation is an increasing clinical problem, but it is uncertain if this is due to inherent lower sensitivity to anthelmintics, reinfestation from the environment, or true anthelmintic resistance.

Onchocerchal dermatitis

Clinical features
- Now uncommon due to use of macrocyclic lactones.
- Hypersensitivity types I and III to microfilariae affecting ventral midline, chest, and withers.
- Pruritus, patchy alopecia, small papules, thickened dry scaly skin, poor hair regrowth, localised particularly to ventral midline.
- In severe cases marked pruritus, excoriation, crusts. Tail rubbing is rare.
- A summer problem. Insects, particularly *Culicoides* spp., act as intermediate hosts.

Diagnosis
- History, signs.
- Biopsy and presence of helminth larvae in affected skin.
- Examination of minced skin, suspended in phosphate-buffered saline for 3 h at 37 °C, filter coarsely, centrifuge for 5 min at 3000 rpm, examine deposit at 60–100x magnification for larvae.
- Differentials: sweet itch, trombiculidiasis. N.B. insect hypersensitivity and onchocerciasis can both be associated with *Culicoides* and so may coexist.

Treatment
- Ivermectin paste (Noromectin, Norbrook; Eraquell, Virbac; Vectin, MSD Animal Health; Eqvalan, Boehringer Animal Health; Animec, Chanelle Pharma; Bimetin, Bimeda) 200-300 µg/kg by mouth or moxidectin gel (Equest, Zoetis UK) 400µg/kg by mouth is effective in killing the larvae. Most cases resolve with one treatment; however, regular treatment is needed as the adult worms are not killed and thus the condition may recur.
- Dying microfilaria may cause acute exacerbation of pruritus in the first 3 days after treatment so concurrent corticosteroids may need to be administered.

Larval nematode dermatitis

Clinical features
- Under unhygienic conditions (muddy yards, contaminated bedding), larvae of the free-living rhabditid nematode, *Pelodera strongyloides*, can invade equine skin and cause irritation.
- Marked pruritus, papules, pustules, ulcers, crusts, alopecia, erythema of limbs, ventrum.

Diagnosis
- Demonstrate motile nematode larvae in skin scrapings; biopsy specimens.

Treatment
- Clean and disinfect skin; can use an antimicrobial cream.
- Clean and rectify environment.
- Signs regress over days to weeks.

MICROBIAL INFECTIONS

Bacterial and fungal infections in which pruritus may be a feature are listed in Table 2.1. These conditions are considered in other sections of the book, as indicated.

Table 2.1 Microbial infections that may feature pruritus

Fungal disease	Causative organism	Bacterial disease	Causative organism
Superficial	Dermatophytes of the genera *Trichophyton* and *Microsporum. Geotrichum candidum.* See Chapter 3.	Folliculitis and furunculosis	Pathogenic staphylococci, streptococci. See Chapter 3.
		Dermatophilosis	*Dermatophilus congolensis.* See Chapter 3.
Deep	e.g. *Drechslera spicifera, Alternaria alternata.* See Chapter 5.	Botryomycosis	See Chapter 5.

Rabies encephalomyelitis

Clinical features

- Rabies is found throughout the world, apart from islands where strict quarantine programmes are in place. The virus mainly affects bats and carnivores, but can affect any mammal.
- In most European and North American countries, the disease is eliminated from domestic animals, although still present in wildlife.
- Horses may be infected by the bite of an infected animal. The incubation period is variable and can be prolonged.
- In the prodromal phase of infection, as the virus spreads by retrograde axonal transport, abnormal sensation around and proximal to the inoculation site may result in pruritic behaviour.
- During the excitation phase, or furious form, affected animals show signs of distress and extreme agitation, often becoming aggressive and unmanageable. Kicking or striking out and rolling may be confused for colic. Self-inflicted wounds may occur.
- The paralytic phase usually involves paralysis of the jaw and throat muscles, causing excessive salivation and inability to swallow. Paralysis spreads and death occurs rapidly.
- Infected animals present a risk of zoonotic transmission.

Diagnosis

- Initial signs are often vague and non-specific, making diagnosis difficult, particularly in areas where rabies is uncommon.
- Where the disease is suspected, euthanasia should be performed and material from the central nervous system submitted for laboratory confirmation.

Treatment
- There is no effective treatment.
- For animals that have been exposed to or bitten by a rabid animal, local guidelines should be followed. For vaccinated horses this is likely to include a rabies booster vaccination and a period of observation. Unvaccinated animals may either be destroyed humanely or undergo a period of extended quarantine.

NON-CONTAGIOUS CONDITIONS

Insect attack

Clinical features
- Insects involved: horse fly (*Tabanus*), stable fly (*Stomoxys*), midges (*Culicoides*), horn fly (*Haematobia*), black fly (*Simulium*), mosquitoes, wasps, bees.
- Signs may include:
  - Crusted papules or wheals at sites of insect bite, presence of a sting, pain, swelling (Figure 2.10).
  - Stamping, restlessness, irritability. Horses may choose to stand in smoke which drives away flies.

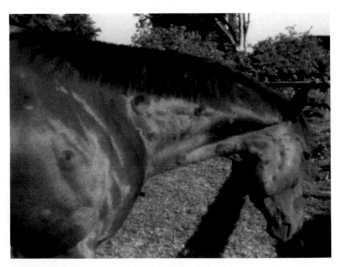

Figure 2.10 Multiple wheals and swellings on the lateral neck and trunk of a horse after attack by a scourge of mosquitoes

Diagnosis
- History, clinical signs, presence of insects.

Treatment
- Depends on severity and pain.
- *Tabanus* and *Stomoxys*:
  - Topical anti-inflammatory or analgesic cream; in severe cases a short-acting systemic glucocorticoid may be needed.
  - Sedation, e.g. acepromazine, 0.08 mg/kg intramuscularly, or by mouth (Sedalin Oral Gel, Vetoquinol) 0.075–0.125 mg/kg to effect; oral detomidine (Domosedan Gel, Zoetis) 40 µg/kg.
- Generally:
  - Repellents and/or persistent insecticides, e.g. synthetic pyrethroids.
  - Change environment – dispose of manure, cut vegetation, use environmental insecticides, depending on the life cycle of the insect(s) responsible, e.g. for *Tabanus*, remove decaying vegetation and manure.

Hypersensitivity disorders
Culicoides hypersensitivity (sweet itch, insect-bite hypersensitivity)

Clinical features
- Worldwide disease occurring in areas where *Culicoides* spp. are found. Populations are promoted by waterlogged ground and low wind speeds. Biting is diurnal and restricted to early morning and late afternoon from early summer to late autumn in the UK. Midges are on the wing when temperatures exceed 12 °C.
- Hypersensitivity occurs principally in horses over 6 months of age, involving Type I and Type IV hypersensitivity reactions against salivary proteins of midges. Familial incidence well recognised.
- Signs occur at insect feeding sites, predominantly the dorsal but also ventral midline, and include:
  - Pruritus indicated by rubbing and the presence of broken hairs, especially in the mane and tail (Figures 2.11 and 2.12).
  - Papules, crusts, exudation, and skin thickening dorsally; lesions occur ventrally (Figure 2.13) where ventrally-feeding species are found.
  - Horses may show irritability, restlessness, and weight loss due to reduced feeding behaviour.

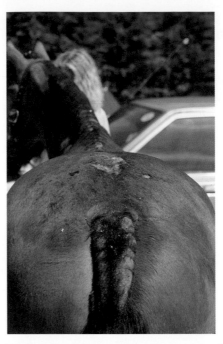

Figure 2.11   Hair loss, crusting, and excoriation affecting the tail and rump in a horse with *Culicoides* hypersensitivity. Hair loss at the withers and of the mane can also be seen.

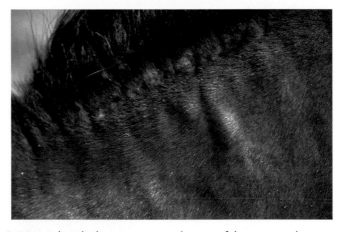

Figure 2.12   *Culicoides* hypersensitivity: alopecia of the mane and crest region with skin thickening and rugal folds.

Diagnosis
- History, signs, presence of midges in the environment.
- Part hair of forelock, mane, and tail to look for feeding midges.

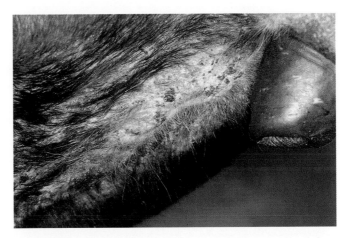

Figure 2.13 Ventral midline alopecia with excoriations, crusted papules, and thickening in a pony with *Culicoides* hypersensitivity.

- Intradermal tests – cross-reaction occurs between different *Culicoides* spp. although less marked with extracts of laboratory-reared midges compared to extracts of wild-type midges native to the affected animal.
- Serological tests for IgE antibodies directed against whole midge extracts are available and tests involving recombinant *Culicoides* salivary proteins are in development.
- Differentials: oxyuriasis, bites or hypersensitivity to other insects, atopic dermatitis (may coexist), contact dermatitis.

Treatment and management
- Prevent access to horses by *Culicoides* spp.:
  - Stable horses from before dusk until after dawn (4 p.m.–8 a.m.).
  - Move away from low-lying pasture, standing water, and woodland.
  - Cover with rugs and hoods (e.g. Boett sweet itch blanket, Rambo sweet itch fly rug, Equi-Theme sweet itch rug).
  - Fine mesh screen for stable windows and doors, or install fans to create a breeze.
- Repellents and insecticides such as cypermethrin (5% concentrate in Deosect 5% Concentrate for Cutaneous Spray, Zoetis; 2.5% in Barricade 'S' Dip and Spray, Zoetis), permethrin (Cooper's Fly Repellent Plus, MSD Animal Health; Dermoline Sweet Itch Lotion, Battles), light oils alone or including citronella (Extra Tail Fly Spray, Pettifer; NAF Off Citronella Wash), DEET (NAF Off Deet Power Equine Fly Repellent).

- Anti-inflammatory and anti-pruritic therapy:
  - Antihistamines have limited effect (none is licensed for use in horses).
  - Prednisolone 0.5–1 mg/kg once daily by mouth until control is achieved, reducing to alternate-day therapy if other measures do not adequately control the problem.
  - Topical soothing creams containing benzyl benzoate also have repellent properties (Benzyl Benzoate Cutaneous Application B.P., Easi-Vet; Killitch Sweet Itch Lotion, Carr & Day & Martin).
  - Herbal spray containing essential oils (Red Healer Equine e Spray, Red Healer Laboratories, Australia).
  - Shampoos containing colloidal oatmeal.
  - Vitamin D3, nicotinamide, (Cavalesse powder for oral solution, Fidavet) may be helpful by reducing histamine production and increasing surface skin lipids.
- Extracts of *Culicoides* are available for inclusion in allergen-specific immunotherapy preparations, but the evidence for benefit is poor with few good clinical trials published. In the future, recombinant *Culicoides* salivary proteins known to be important in the aetiopathology of the disease may become available for immunotherapy.
- On a welfare basis, the use of electric fencing cannot be condoned as this does nothing to relieve the underlying pruritus, but merely inflicts a more unpleasant sensation than the primary disease.

Atopic dermatitis

Clinical features
- Hypersensitivity reactions to a wide variety of environmental agents including dust and forage mites, pollens, and moulds.
- Signs:
  - Recurrent pruritus and/or urticaria (Figures 2.14, 2.15); variable seasonality.
  - Secondary lesions of alopecia, excoriation, scaling, lichenification, skin thickening, hyperpigmentation.

Diagnosis
- History, signs.
- Rule out other pruritic diseases.
- Intradermal tests (Figure 2.16).
- Serological tests for circulating IgE offered by several commercial laboratories, using a variety of reagents to demonstrate allergen-specific equine IgE, including polyclonal antisera; monoclonal

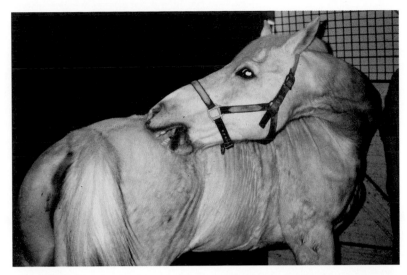

Figure 2.14 Intense pruritus in a horse with atopic dermatitis, intradermal test positive to indoor (stable) allergens.

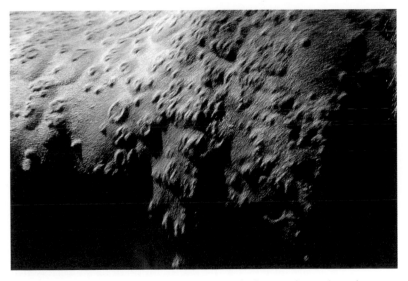

Figure 2.15 Urticaria in an atopic horse: multiple raised papules, plaques, and annular lesions on the trunk and shoulder region.

anti-equine IgE antibodies, single or mixed; modified recombinant high-affinity Fc-receptor peptide (Allercept reagent, Heska). Note poor inter-assay correlation and poor to no correlation with intra-dermal test results.
- Biopsy not particularly helpful as it shows a non-specific superficial perivascular dermatitis, predominantly eosinophilic.

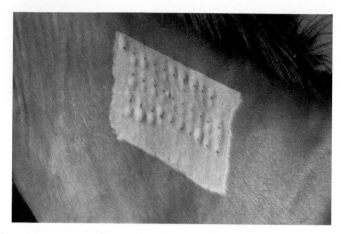

Figure 2.16 Intradermal tests in an atopic horse.

- Differentials: insect-bite hypersensitivity, oxyuriasis, *Malassezia* dermatitis, contact dermatitis, food sensitivity.

Treatment and management
- Allergen avoidance, e.g. remove bedding material, thoroughly clean stable, maintain at pasture.
- Anti-pruritic therapy:
  - Prednisolone 0.5–1 mg/kg once daily by mouth until control is achieved, then reduce to lowest alternate-day regimen. Alternatively, dexamethasone short-acting injection (Dexa-Ject, Bimeda; Duphacort Q, Zoetis; Dexadreson, MSD Animal Health, Colvasone, Norbrook Laboratories; Rapidexon, Dechra) 0.01–0.02 mg/kg intramuscularly as a loading dose, followed by oral prednisolone or use of dexamethasone tablets (Dexacortone, Dechra Veterinary Products, off-label use) 0.02–0.1 mg/kg by mouth every 48–72 h.
  - Antihistamines: none is licensed for veterinary use, but the following tablets may be useful alone or as steroid-sparing agents:
    - Hydroxyzine (Atarax, Pfizer) 0.5–2 mg/kg twice or three times daily.
    - Chlorphenamine (Piriton, Allercalm, Hayleve) 0.25–0.5 mg/kg twice or three times daily.
    - Diphenhydramine (Nytol capsules) 1–2 mg/kg twice or three times daily.
    - Alimemazine, formerly trimeprazine (Zentiva) 1–2 mg/kg twice or three times daily.
    - Cetirizine (Zyrtec) 0.2–0.4 mg/kg twice daily.

- Tricyclic antidepressants (not licensed for veterinary use) such as amitriptyline 1 mg/kg twice daily by mouth can be helpful in chronic pruritus by potentiating the effect of other anti-pruritic drugs and antihistaminic effects.
    - Milk casein-derived nutraceuticals (e.g. Calmex Equine, VetPlus; Zylkene Equine, Vetoquinol) may be helpful for reducing anxiety and stress that can exacerbate pruritus.
- Allergen-specific immunotherapy based on intradermal test results is reported to be beneficial in 65–85% of cases.
- Essential fatty acids do not seem useful generally but anecdotally may help some horses.
- Some cases prove to be highly refractive to treatment.

Adverse food reactions

Clinical features
- A rare and poorly documented disease, no case series in the literature.
- May cause urticaria and pruritus; telogen defluxion has also been reported.
- Diagnosis is often suspected but rarely confirmed.

Diagnosis
- Exclude other urticarial and pruritic diseases.
- Carry out a food exclusion trial, e.g. with grass pellets and single species hay or wilted grass product for at least a month.
- Confirm by provocative challenge and subsequent improvement again when suspect food is discontinued.

Treatment and management
- Change diet.

Contact dermatitis

- See Chapter 3.

Malassezia dermatitis

Clinical features
- *Malassezia* spp. are found as normal commensals at carriage sites such as the ear, nose, intermammary region, and preputial fossa of healthy horses, but have been found in large numbers in mares with pruritus associated with intermammary dermatitis ('cleavage itch'); occasionally

found in large numbers in lesions of self-induced alopecia on other areas of the body (Figure 2.17). Although not yet proven in the horse, hypersensitivity may be involved in the aetiology in affected animals.

- Signs in intermammary *Malassezia* dermatitis include kicking at belly, rubbing the tail – both dorsal and ventral aspects, dragging belly on the ground whilst rolling. Greasy brown exudate is present in the intertriginous regions.
- Elsewhere on the body, it may cause alopecia, erythema, excoriations, scaling.

Diagnosis

- Demonstration of large numbers of monopolar budding yeast organisms on cytological samples.
- Differentials: oxyuriasis, insect-bite hypersensitivity, atopic dermatitis, contact dermatitis.

Treatment

- Clean with shampoo containing ingredient(s) effective against yeast organisms, e.g. chlorhexidine, chloroxylenol, acetic acid, selenium sulphide, azole drugs.
- Topical application of antifungal preparations: none licensed for equine use, but small animal products such as miconazole nitrate with prednisolone and polymyxin B (Surolan Ear Drops and Cutaneous Suspension,

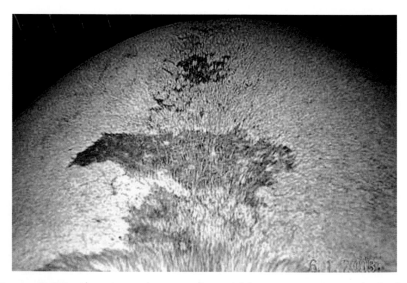

Figure 2.17 Alopecia, erythema, scaling, and hyperpigmentation on the lumbar region associated with large numbers of yeast organisms, which resolved with topical antifungal therapy.

Elanco) or human products such as clotrimazole (Canesten, Bayer; various generic brands) or miconazole (Daktarin, Janssen-Cilag; various generic brands) once daily until resolution of dermatitis and pruritus.
- Ongoing regular cleaning of carriage areas as part of routine grooming regime.

Immune-mediated disease

Some cases of pemphigus foliaceous present with marked generalised pruritus. See Chapter 3.

Neoplasia

Generalised pruritus may be a feature of mast cell tumours. See Chapter 5.

Neurogenic pruritus
Post-traumatic dysaesthesia

Clinical features
- Damage to the spinal cord may result in altered cutaneous sensory perception (dysaesthesia).
- Excessive pruritic behaviour, including rubbing and scratching with hind feet, has been documented in horses that have sustained cervical spinal injuries.
- The abnormal sensation and response are usually restricted to the dermatome(s) affected by the neurological damage; occasionally localised hyperhidrosis is also seen.
- Skin changes when present are due to self-inflicted trauma.

Diagnosis
- History of cervical spinal trauma.
- Absence of primary skin lesions.
- Radiographic imaging of cervical spine.

Treatment
- Depends on nature of lesion and concurrent neurological signs:
  - Conservative management with use of non-steroidal anti-inflammatory therapy may result in improvement in time.
  - Euthanasia on humane grounds may be indicated.

REFERENCES AND FURTHER READING

Cox, A., Wood, K., Coleman, G. et al. (2020) Essential oil spray reduces clinical signs of insect-bite hypersensitivity in horses. *Australian Veterinary Journal*, 98: 411–416.

Da Silva, A.S., Tonin, A., and Lopes, L.S. (2013) Outbreak of lice in horses: Epidemiology, diagnosis, and treatment. *Journal of Equine Veterinary Science*, 33: 530–532.

Loeffler. A., Herrick, D., Allen, S. et al. (2018) Long-term management of horses with atopic dermatitis in southeastern England: A retrospective questionnaire study of owners' perceptions. *Veterinary Dermatology*, 29: 526–533-e176.

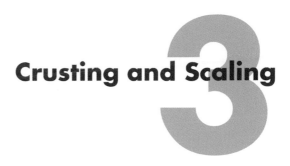

Crusting and Scaling

IDIOPATHIC SEBORRHOEIC CONDITIONS

There are several clinical syndromes where excessive scaling is the primary presenting sign, with no underlying disease evident. There is probably an underlying abnormality of cornification in these cases, i.e. a primary keratinisation defect, which thus far has not been fully characterised.

Mane and tail seborrhoea

Clinical features
- An uncommon disorder characterised by moderate to severe scaling in the mane and, or, tail regions (Figure 3.1).
- No age, breed, or sex predilections reported.
- Scaling may be dry or oily, and rafts of scale may be adherent to the skin surface.
- There is little or no accompanying pruritus, but there may be some alopecia of the tail.

Diagnosis
- Signs, rule out other possible causes such as selenosis.

Practical Equine Dermatology, Second Edition. Janet D. Littlewood, David H. Lloyd and J. Mark Craig.
© 2022 John Wiley & Sons Ltd. Published 2022 by John Wiley & Sons Ltd.

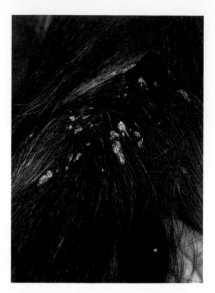

Figure 3.1 Tail seborrhoea in a young thoroughbred colt. Large flakes of desquamated corneocytes visible.

Treatment
- Symptomatic treatment consisting of frequent, regular use of antiseborrhoeic, keratoplastic shampoo or sprays: products marketed for small animals containing ingredients such as colloidal sulphur and salicylates (e.g. Coatex Medicated Shampoo, Vet Plus; Malabeze, Forte Healthcare; Sebomild, Virbac; Zincoseb Shampoo or Spray, Vetruus), coal tar, and sulphur (Johnsons Skin Calm Shampoo); 1% selenium sulphide shampoo (veterinary product Seleen no longer available; human equivalent Selsun Blue, Sanofi; note that human product Selsun, Delpharm Bladel B.V., is 2.5% concentration) or coal tar shampoos. Lotions or creams containing organic acids (e.g. Dermisol Cream, Zoetis UK) can be used prior to or in between shampoo washes to facilitate scale removal.
- Application of humectants conditioners or moisturisers (Humilac, Virbac; Ermidra Spray or Foam, Vetruus) may be beneficial as a rinse after, and between, bathing.

Generalised seborrhoea

Clinical features
- A rare scaling disorder. Both dry and oily forms may be seen. Extremities tend to be spared.
- Non-pruritic unless secondary bacterial or yeast infection are present.

Diagnosis
- Rule out all causes of secondary seborrhoea.

Treatment
- Symptomatic, as above.

Mallenders and Sallenders

Clinical features
- Condition characterised by hyperkeratosis and scaling on the palmar aspects of the carpi (mallenders) and, or, anterior aspects of the tarsi (sallenders) seen in cob and heavy horse breeds (Figure 3.2).
- May develop fissures and secondary bacterial and, or, yeast infection, which may be variably pruritic.

Diagnosis
- Signs, tape strips, and surface scrapings for microscopical examination to rule out chorioptic mange mites and identify secondary infections.

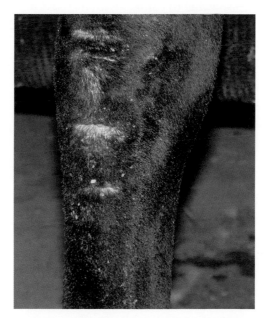

Figure 3.2 Mallenders. Horizontal linear crusting and scaling on palmar aspect of carpus of a cob; this case was associated with secondary *Malassezia* dermatitis.

Treatment
- Topical therapy as above, with additional antimicrobial activity if appropriate (e.g. Coatex Medicated Shampoo, Vet Plus; Malabeze, Forte Healthcare; Zincoseb shampoo, Vetruus; Sebomild P, Sebolytic Shampoo, Sebomild Lotion, Virbac).

SECONDARY, ACQUIRED KERATINISATION AND CRUSTING DISORDERS

INFECTIOUS CAUSES

Superficial fungal infections

Dermatophytosis

Clinical features
- Over-diagnosed; clinical diagnosis is often based on presenting signs, which can be deceptive. May occur sporadically in outbreaks. Predominantly affects young horses.
- Several species of dermatophyte may cause disease:
  - *Trichophyton equinum* var. *equinum* is the most common aetiological agent; infections with *T. mentagrophytes* and *T. verrucosum* may occur due to contact with infected reservoir hosts.
    - Incubation period usually about 10 days, but may be up to 4 weeks.
    - Can be very pruritic especially in "girth itch". A scratch reflex can often be elicited.
    - Spontaneous recovery generally occurs in 5–6 weeks, but lesions may be prolonged if a secondary bacterial infection is present. Course is generally longer in horses under 4 years old.
  - *Microsporum equinum*:
    - Causes a milder syndrome than *T. equinum* and *T. mentagrophytes*.
    - Sometimes wrongly identified as *M. canis*.
  - *Microsporum gypseum*:
    - Usually less severe, less pruritic, and more focal than other dermatophytes, but may be more widespread.
    - Can be transmitted by tabanid flies.
  - Other dermatophytes may occasionally cause disease.
- Early lesions may resemble urticaria. Lesions tend to be localised and focal or multifocal. Erythema may be visible in non-pigmented skin. Hairs are typically raised; lesions extend peripherally.

- Scaling, crusting, and hair loss develop (Figures 3.3 and 3.4). Crusts may be quite thick (5 mm) and can be grossly indistinguishable from those of dermatophilosis; however, *Dermatophilus congolensis* does not damage the hair shafts. On recovery, hair growth usually starts at the centre of lesions.
- Pruritus is variable.

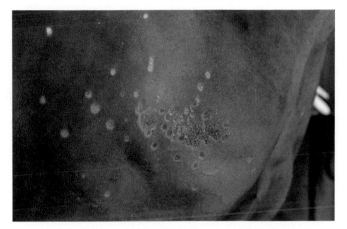

Figure 3.3 *Trichophyton* infection. Multiple annular lesions of scaling, crusting, and alopecia.

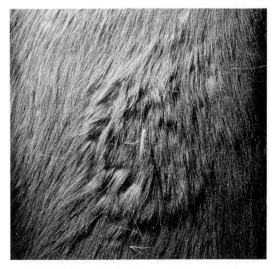

Figure 3.4 Crusted lesions with hair tufts in a case of *Trichophyton equinum* infection. Source: Courtesy of Veterinary Record.

Diagnosis

- History, especially evidence of transmission to and, or, from other animals or humans.
- Signs.
- Confirmation:
  - Examine crusts and hairs. Rule out dermatophilosis (impression smears). Demonstrate arthroconidia (arthrospores) and, or, hyphae.
  - Collect crusts and hairs for dermatophyte culture and species identification. Note that *T. equinum* var. *equinum* has a specific requirement for niacin which may need to be added to the culture medium.
  - More rapid confirmation of infection can be obtained with special staining of skin biopsies.
  - Hairs infected with *M. equinum* exhibit yellow-green fluorescence under the Wood's lamp.
  - Differentials: dermatophilosis, staphylococcal folliculitis, pemphigus foliaceus.

Treatment

- Spontaneous recovery makes assessment of the efficacy of therapy difficult.
- No systemic antifungal agents are licensed for use in the horse. Published studies of clinical studies with griseofulvin in equine dermatophytosis are flawed.
- Topical therapies include:
  - Enilconazole (Imaverol, Janssen); wash with 0.2% solution every 3 days on four occasions.
  - Miconazole 2% and chlorhexidine 2% shampoo (Malaseb, Dechra), licensed for dogs, has been shown to be effective in horses; affected animals were bathed twice weekly, asymptomatic in-contact animals once weekly. No active lesions seen after 4 weeks; treatment discontinued after 5 weeks.
  - Sulphurated lime (1:40 dilution of Lime Sulphur Dip, Easi-Vet; 1 in 32 dilution of Lime Sulfur Dip, Vetoquinol USA) applied as a leave-on rinse, daily for 5–7 days then once or twice weekly until clinical cure.
- Spores can survive for months on hair shafts and in crusts, and topical therapy is unlikely to kill all arthrospores within hair follicles, necessitating repeated treatments as infected hairs grow out.
- Efficacy of therapy should be checked by clinical examination for lesion resolution, and by sampling (Mackenzie brush technique useful) for fungal culture.

Control
- Spores can remain viable in stable environment and grooming equipment for months to years.
- Isolate infected animals to prevent transmission to other animals and people.
- Disinfect accommodation, boxes, tack. Identify and eliminate sources of infection.
- Treat tack, grooming items, and environment with imidazole foggers (imazalil in PacRite Fungaflor, Pace), or with potassium monopersulphate sprays (Virkon, Lanxess) to reduce contamination.

Dermatomycosis – Geotrichosis

Clinical features
- Cutaneous infection with the yeast-like organism *Geotrichum candidum*, commonly found in the environment, can cause very similar signs to dermatophytosis.
- Signs:
  - Annular to patchy alopecia, particularly affecting head and neck.
  - Most cases also show scaling.
  - A third of cases are pruritic.

Diagnosis
- Signs.
- Microscopical examination of crusts, hair plucks, surface adhesive tape strips.
- Fungal culture.
- Differentials – dermatophytosis.

Treatment
- Topical antifungal therapy.
  - Resolution of clinical signs documented after one month of treatment with antifungal disinfectant containing bleach.
  - Products listed above for dermatophytosis would also be expected to be effective.

Bacterial infections

Dermatophilosis

Clinical features
- Infection with *Dermatophilus congolensis* requires presence of zoospores, which can survive for many months in crusts and shorter

periods in moist soil, together with moisture and damage to the epidermal barrier.

- Two main clinical syndromes:
  - 'Rain scald' affecting the dorso-lateral trunk, at sites of water run-off.
  - 'Mud fever' affecting the distal limbs, one of the differentials/contributory factors to "greasy heel" syndrome (Figure 3.5). The organism appears to be less frequently involved as a cause of pastern dermatitis than once thought.
  - Less commonly, lesions may occur elsewhere, including face and muzzle.
- Generally, occurs in wet weather, especially autumn and winter, and following prolonged and, or, heavy rain.
- Trauma to the skin predisposes to infection, e.g. grooming, clipping, sharp vegetation.
- Non-pigmented skin is predisposed.
- Recurs in previously affected horses, and may spread to in-contact animals; presence of sheep with lumpy wool can be a source of infective zoospores.
- Lesion development:
  - Focal, tufted, paintbrush lesions progress into thick crusts (Figures 3.6 and 3.7), with a concave undersurface covered by a thin layer of pus.

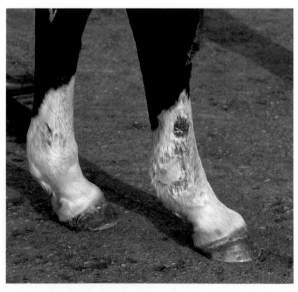

Figure 3.5 Dermatophilosis. Erythema, crusting, and alopecia in the white-haired lateral and medial surfaces of the hind limbs.

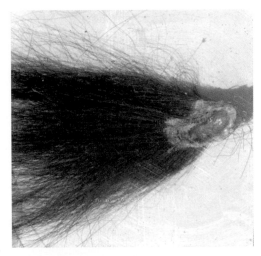

Figure 3.6 Thick scab with attached hair from a lesion of dermatophilosis. Note the concave surface covered with purulent exudate.

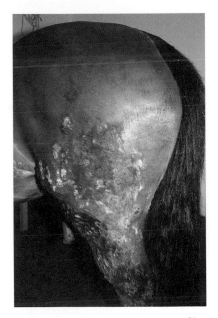

Figure 3.7 Dermatophilosis. Raised crusts and matting of hair, patchy alopecia, and areas of ulceration with haemorrhagic and purulent exudation.

– Long coats may disguise the extent of lesions.
– Hairs are not damaged, but are epilated leading to alopecia when crusts are removed.
– In wet areas, the crusts may not remain attached. Prolonged wetting of the skin leading to maceration may allow secondary infec-

tion. When this involves the limbs, it may result in oedema and cellulitis.

- Human infection can occur, and hygienic precautions should be taken.

Diagnosis

- History, signs, impression smears (Gram or Giemsa stain). The appearance of *Dermatophilus* is diagnostic (Gram-positive, branching filaments breaking up into multiple rows of cocci, "train-track" appearance; Figure 3.8). The vigorously motile zoospores may be visible in crushed scabs emulsified in water or saline).
- Material from crusts can be cultured, but it can be difficult to isolate the slow-growing *Dermatophilus;* increased carbon dioxide in culture environment facilitates growth.
- Polymerase chain reaction (PCR) assays are now available to detect *Dermatophilus* infection.
- Differentials: dermatophytosis, bacterial folliculitis, other causes of greasy heel – pastern dermatitis, photosensitisation, contact dermatitis, leucocytoclastic vasculitis.

Treatment

- Bring in to dry housing.
- Remove crusts manually or with keratolytic rinses, creams, or shampoos (Dermisol cream or lotion, Zoetis UK; salicylates + sodium thiosulphate with chloroxylenol in Coatex Medicated Shampoo, VetPlus

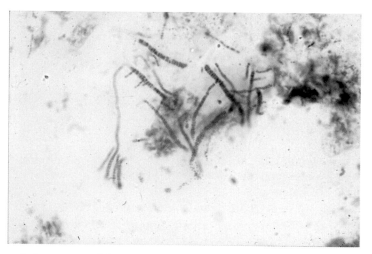

Figure 3.8 Dermatophilosis. Giemsa-stained smear from an emulsified scab. Note the characteristic branching filaments composed of parallel rows of cocci.

or Malabeze, Forte Healthcare; salicylates with chlorhexidine in Zincoseb, Vetruus); hairs remain attached to the crusts and may need to be cut to aid detachment. Sedation may be necessary.

- Dispose of crusts carefully, as they are a source of new infection; use a dedicated area for washing that can be properly disinfected.
- Wash daily with topical antibacterial agents, e.g. chlorhexidine shampoos or scrubs, diluted to 1–2%, or other small animal medicated shampoos as above, with 5–10 minutes contact time with lather, rinse, and dry well. If daily washing is not possible then chlorhexidine mousse or sprays marketed for small animals can be applied on the intervening days, without rinsing off (e.g. Douxo S3 Pyo Mousse; Clorexyderm spray or foam, Vetruus).
- The humectant and antibacterial combination of glycols, alcohols, and triclosan has been shown to be effective in mud fever cases, by limiting water activity required by bacterial organisms (Mud Stop Antibacterial Spray, Antibacterial Gel, Disinfectant Cream, Equitech).
- Chlorine-based products can also be used in the control of mud fever and can be used prophylactically (e.g. Equi-Oxcide Treatment and Barrier Spray, Trus-Steed; Vetericyn VF Spray, Innovacyn).
- Topical antibiotics such as silver sulphadiazine (Flamazine, Smith & Nephew), neomycin, polymyxin B, fusidic acid in various small animal topical ear or skin lotion products.
- Systemic antibiotics may be needed in severe cases or when other infections are involved. Systemic treatment allows healing at the skin surface and separation of the crusts which can then be more easily removed. *Dermatophilus* is usually sensitive to first-level antibiotics such as trimethoprim-potentiated sulphadiazine (Trimediazine Powder/Oral Paste, Vetoquinol; Norodine Equine Oral Paste, Norbrook) 30 mg/kg by mouth every 12 hours, or procaine penicillin with dihydrostreptomycin (Pen & Strep Suspension for Injection, Norbrook Laboratories) at a dose of 1 ml per 12.5 kg once daily (higher than labelled dose to comply with recommended guidelines for responsible antimicrobial usage). Antibiosis should continue until infection has completely resolved.
- Lesions on the distal limbs can be very painful. Pain and inflammation may be relieved by the use of topical glucocorticoid creams, in conjunction with topical antibiotics.
- Isolate affected animals, and disinfect tack and grooming kit to avoid spread to other animals and humans. Most disinfectants will readily kill *Dermatophilus*. Rugs and saddle cloths should be washed with biocidal detergent or additive (e.g. Trus-Steed Biocidal Rug Wash).
- Advise owners regarding risk of recurrence in future periods of wet weather, and use of topical antiseptics on a prophylactic basis.

Superficial folliculitis and furunculosis

Clinical features

- Most commonly associated with infection involving *Staphylococcus aureus*, but other pathogenic staphylococci such as *S. pseudintermedius*, *S. hyicus*, and streptococcal organisms may also be involved.
- Localised syndromes:
  - Truncal folliculitis affecting the saddle region, other areas of tack, or rider's boot contact, often occurring at the time of change of coat, in spring, or associated with clipping in the late autumn/winter.
  - Pastern folliculitis affecting the caudolateral aspects of distal limbs. Non-pigmented limbs predisposed.
  - Tail pyoderma, due to secondary infection following cutaneous trauma produced by tail rubbing.
- Lesions consist of folliculocentric papules which may develop into pustules, oedema, exudation, and crusting, with focal alopecia when hairs are lost from infected follicles (Figures 3.9 and 3.10).
- May progress to furunculosis and occasionally formation of abscesses; swelling of limbs due to cellulitis is sometimes seen. In long-standing or complicated cases, opportunistic mixed infections involving Gram-negative and anaerobic organisms may be seen. Usually, painful rather than pruritic.
- Ill-fitting tack and poor hygiene as well as non-pigmented skin may be predisposing factors. Outbreaks can occur in groups of horses, particularly where tack and grooming items are shared.

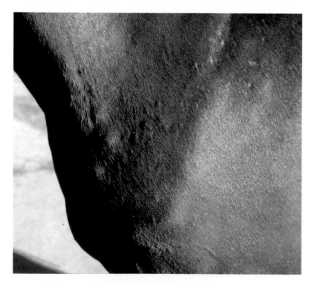

Figure 3.9 Staphylococcal folliculitis and furunculosis.

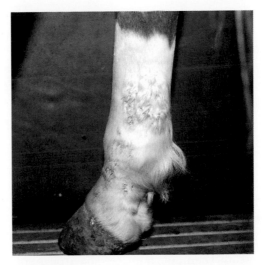

Figure 3.10 Bacterial folliculitis of pastern and metatarsal regions. Staphylococci and streptococci were isolated.

- Reports of meticillin-resistant organisms are becoming more common, and there is increasing evidence of transfer of meticillin-resistant *S. aureus* (MRSA) amongst horses and veterinary staff, and of carriage of livestock-associated MRSA CC398 by horses.

Diagnosis
- Signs.
- Microscopical examination of impression smears of lesions or the underside of crusts or emulsified crusts reveal presence of bacterial cocci with neutrophils and inflammatory cell debris.
- Bacterial culture and sensitivity testing is indicated in cases not responding to logical empirical treatment or where animals have received systemic antibiotics previously. Surface swab samples may not be representative, and material from deep within lesions or biopsy material is recommended for bacterial isolation.
- Differentials: dermatophytosis, dermatophilosis, other causes of greasy heel syndrome.

Treatment
- Wash daily with antiseptic or medicated shampoo for about 7 days and then twice weekly until resolution:
  - Chlorhexidine 4% in surgical scrub (Hibiscrub Medical, Mölnlycke Healthcare; Vetasept, Animal Care Group; Vet-Hands, VetWay) or in shampoos marketed for small animals (Clorexyderm, Vetruus;

Microbex, Virbac) with ophytrium (Douxo S3 Pyo shampoo, Ceva), with miconazole (Malaseb, Dechra Veterinary Products), or with keratoplastic agents (Zincoseb, Vetruus). Dilute approximately 1 in 4, lather and cleanse lesions to remove crusts, allow 10 minutes contact time then rinse thoroughly.

– Other small animal shampoos include chloroxylenol with keratoplastic agents (Coatex Medicated Shampoo, VetPlus; Malabeze, Forte Healthcare), which needs only 5 minutes contact time, and ethyl lactate (Etiderm, Virbac).

• Antiseptic spray, mousse, or gel (Douxo S3 Pyo Mousse, Ceva; Clorexyderm Spray, Foam, Gel, Vetruus) can be used between shampoos and prophylactically, as can chlorine-based antiseptic sprays as described for dermatophilosis. Antiseptic and humectant combinations of glycols, alcohols, and triclosan in the Mud Stop range (spray, gel, cream, shampoo; EquiTech) have been shown to be effective in cases of pastern dermatitis associated with various bacterial infections.

• Topical antibiotics in conjunction with glucocorticoids in products licensed for small animals may be useful for localised lesions e.g. fusidic acid (Isaderm Gel, Dechra Veterinary Products; Betafuse, Norbrook Laboratories), polymyxin B (Surolan Cutaneous Suspension, Elanco UK AH), or gentamicin (Otomax Ear Drops, MSD Animal Health; Easotic, Virbac).

• Systemic antibiotics in severe cases or where topical therapy alone fails to secure resolution. First-line antibiotics should always be selected in the first instance; treatment should continue beyond clinical cure (usually at least 3 weeks), alongside ongoing topical therapy. (See BEVA resources for vets Protect ME antimicrobial policy guidance, www. beva.org.uk//Portals/0/Documents/ResourcesForVets/1beva-antimicrobial-policy-template-distributed.pdf.). The doses recommended below are as advised in the literature and in the guidance document, rather than those stated in the data sheets:

– First-line antibiotic choice is trimethoprim-potentiated sulphadiazine (Trimediazine Powder/Oral Paste, Vetoquinol; Norodine Equine Oral Paste, Norbrook Laboratories) 30 mg/kg by mouth twice daily, every 12 hours.

– Alternative choice is off-label use of doxycycline solution (Karidox 100 mg/ml solution for chicken and pigs, Nimrod Veterinary Products)10 mg/kg by mouth every 12 hours.

– Injectable alternatives include procaine penicillin (Depocillin 300 mg/ml solution, MSD Animal Health) 20,000–25,000 iu/kg (12–15 mg/kg) intramuscularly every 12 hours, or with dihydrostreptomycin 20 mg/kg intramuscularly every 24 hours (Pen & Strep Suspension for Injection, Norbrook Laboratories; dose of

1 ml per 12.5 kg bodyweight); or gentamicin (Genta-Equine 100 mg/ml solution for injection, Dechra Veterinary Products) 6.6 mg/kg intravenously every 24 hours.
- Second-level antibiotics such as fluoroquinolones and third-generation cephalosporins should be protected and only used on the basis of culture and sensitivity when there are no suitable first- or second-line options. When deemed necessary, either ceftiofur (Excenel, Zoetis UK) 2 mg/kg intramuscularly every 12 hours, or off-label cefquinome (Cobactan 25 mg/ml suspension for injection, MSD Animal Health) 1 mg/kg intramuscularly every 24 hours can be given. Off-label enrofloxacin 100 mg/ml solution for poultry can be given orally (Baytril 10% Oral Solution, Elanco; Lanflox 100 mg/ml solution, Nimrod; Enroxil 100 mg/ml solution, Dechra) at a dose of 7.5 mg/kg once daily.
- Disinfect tack, rugs, grooming items thoroughly. Correct any management problems. Identify and eliminate sources of infection.

Mucocutaneous pyoderma

Clinical features
- Occasionally, staphylococcal infection may be restricted to mucocutaneous areas, particularly periorally (Figure 3.11) and sometimes periocularly.
- Initiating factors unclear, but likely to involve local trauma.
- Erythema, ulceration, exudation, crusting, and depigmentation.

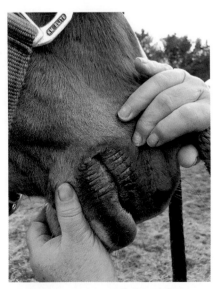

Figure 3.11 Mucocutaneous pyoderma affecting the lips and perioral area. Source: Courtesy of Ewan Macaulay.

Diagnosis
- Signs, microscopical examination of surface impressions, or tape strips to confirm presence of bacterial cocci, and inflammatory cells and cellular debris.

Treatment
- Topical antiseptics and antibiotics as described above for folliculitis and furunculosis in the first instance.
- Systemic antibiotics if failing to resolve with topical therapy.

Viral infections
Aural plaques

See Chapter 5.

Occult sarcoids

See Chapter 5.

IMMUNE-MEDIATED CAUSES

Pemphigus foliaceus

Clinical features
- Commonest of the autoimmune skin diseases of equidae.
- Antibodies directed against epidermal cell surface antigens result in loss of intercellular cohesion and the formation of intraepidermal vesicles or, more usually, vesicopustules.
- No sex predisposition.
- Age of onset is important with respect to the prognosis. Cases in animals less than one year of age tend to be less severe, respond well to therapy, and may spontaneously regress.

Signs
- Whilst the primary lesion is a vesicle or vesicopustule, the usual presentation is a crusting, scaling dermatosis that often begins on the face, but commonly becomes generalised (Figures 3.12 and 3.13).
- In some cases, in older horses, lesions are limited to the coronary band (Figure 3.14), chestnut, and ergot regions, and occasionally the frog.
- Intact vesicles are hard to find. Lesions consist of areas of focal crusting, annular erosions, and alopecia.

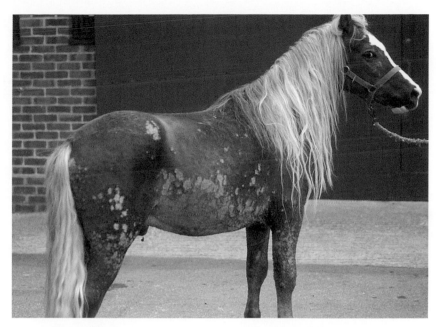

Figure 3.12 Generalised crusting and coalescing annular alopecia in a stallion with pemphigus foliaceous.

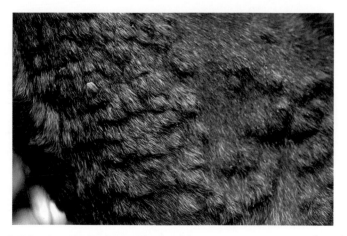

Figure 3.13 Crusting and matted tufts of hair in a young pony with widespread lesions of pemphigus foliaceous.

- Oedema of the extremities and ventrum may be present, often out of proportion to the surface skin changes. Although mucocutaneous sites are often involved, the mucosal surfaces are rarely affected.
- Concurrent systemic signs of fever, depression, and anorexia are seen in severe cases.

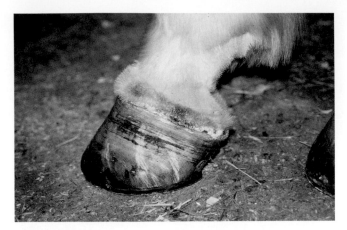

Figure 3.14 Crusting and haemorrhagic erosion and ulceration affecting the coronary band of a 14-year-old horse with pemphigus foliaceous.

- Pruritus is absent to variable, but can be marked.
- Ultraviolet light exposure may exacerbate lesions.

Diagnosis
- Diagnostic investigations should include microscopical examination of vesicle or pustule contents, surface impressions of recently ruptured lesions, and crusts, looking for acantholytic cells; bacterial and fungal culture; and multiple skin biopsies, including crusts, for histopathological examination.
- Cytological examination of vesicle or pustule contents, or impression smears from a recently ruptured vesicopustule or underside of crust, reveals the presence of acantholytic keratinocytes and non-degenerative neutrophils and, or, eosinophils with an absence of bacteria (unless there is surface contamination after rupture of the primary lesion).
- Histologically the primary lesion is an intraepidermal or subcorneal vesicopustule containing acantholytic cells together with neutrophils and sometimes eosinophils, which may predominate.
- Lesions are fragile and transient, and the only clue to the diagnosis may be the presence of large numbers of acantholytic keratinocytes in the surface crusts.
- Auto-antibodies can be demonstrated by direct immunofluorescence or immunohistochemical techniques in 50–75% cases which have not received corticosteroids.
- Differentials: dermatophilosis, dermatophytosis, superficial folliculitis, generalised granulomatous disease, idiopathic seborrhoea.

Treatment

- The disease in young horses usually carries a good prognosis, and treatment can secure lifelong remission; however, some cases fail to respond.
- In older horses, even though the initial response to treatment may be good, permanent maintenance therapy is required. Remission may not be achieved and so the prognosis remains guarded to fair.
- Immunosuppressive therapy should not be employed without confirmation of the diagnosis. Owners should be made aware of the need for lifelong therapy, and the nature and expense of the drugs involved, at the outset. Remission may not be achieved in both older and younger horses, so prognosis remains guarded.
- Corticosteroids are the treatment of choice:
  - Either prednisolone at a dose of 2–4 mg/kg once daily by mouth or a loading dose of dexamethasone (Dexa-Ject 2 mg/ml solution, Bimeda; Duphacort Q 0.2% w/v solution, Zoetis UK; Dexadreson 2 mg/ml solution, MSD Animal Health; Colvasone 0.2% w/v solution, Norbrook Laboratories; Rapidexon 2 mg/ml solution, Dechra Veterinary Products) 0.2 mg/kg by injection. Oral dexamethasone tablets for ongoing treatment (Dexacortone, Dechra Veterinary Products, off-label use) can be given at a dose rate of 0.2–0.4 mg/kg.
  - Marked clinical improvement is usually seen within 10–14 days. At this stage, as long as no new lesions are appearing, the dose of steroids can be gradually reduced.
  - Several protocols exist for tapering the dose of steroids, but too rapid reduction can result in recurrence of lesions, which may be hard to get back into remission.
  - To reduce potential side effects, rather than reducing the daily dose to the lowest possible maintenance dose and then doubling to give on alternate days, reduction of the dose on an alternate-day basis is advisable as soon as the condition is inactive. The dose on alternate days is reduced by 40–50%, keeping the initial dose on the intervening day (i.e. dose reduction of 20–25% over a 48-hour period). Reductions of the alternate-day dose should be made every 2 weeks, with gradual withdrawal leaving the horse on alternate-day dosing. It may be possible to reduce further the alternate-day dose to the lowest possible maintenance dose.
  - Whilst steroids at anti-inflammatory dose rates have not been shown to be associated with an increased risk of laminitis, the

higher dose required for immunosuppression may be associated with potential risk, and owners should be warned. Horses with a history of laminitis or at risk because of high body condition scores may not be suitable for this treatment.

- For cases that fail to respond to corticosteroids or when the dose required to maintain remission is unacceptably high, or when corticosteroids are contraindicated, combination therapy or single therapy with the following can be employed.
  - ◦ Azathioprine (no veterinary licensed product) at a dose of 2–3 mg/kg by mouth every 24 hours to induce remission then every 48 hours for maintenance.
  - ◦ Gold therapy, previously used for management of rheumatoid arthritis in people, has been used successfully in the treatment of pemphigus foliaceus, but manufacture of sodium aurothiomalate has been discontinued, and no alternatives are available in the UK.
- Topical symptomatic therapy with both antiseptic and keratoplastic products to aid in resolution of crusts and control of surface microbial populations should be employed.

Cutaneous lupus erythematosus

Clinical features

- Classically, lupus erythematosus is divided into two forms, chronic cutaneous lupus erythematosus involving the skin and occasionally the mucous membranes, and systemic lupus erythematosus (SLE), which is a multisystemic disease with frequent skin involvement.
- Cutaneous signs and dermatohistopathology of the chronic cutaneous form and SLE in the horse are similar, and thus the disease may be best referred to as cutaneous lupus erythematosus (CLE).
- CLE is relatively rare and cases with systemic involvement are very rare. Various factors including genetic predisposition, ultraviolet light exposure, immune dysfunction, viral infections, hormones, and drugs may be involved in the aetiology.
- Usually occurs in adult horses with no known breed or sex predilection.
- Signs:
  - Major sign is depigmentation with patchy alopecia and varying degrees of erythema and scaling.
  - Lesions commonly found on the face, around the eyes, lips, and nostrils (Figure 3.15); perianal and genital areas may also be

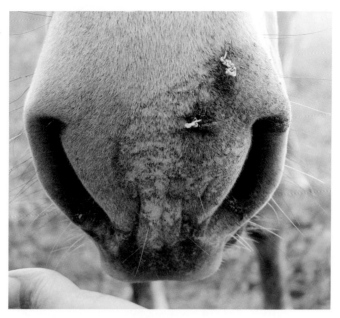

Figure 3.15 Cutaneous lupus erythematosus. Asymmetric patchy depigmentation with erythema and mild crusting affecting the muzzle, left external nares, and upper lip. Sutures are present at biopsy sites.

involved. In long-standing cases, there is thickening and the skin may appear like "wrinkled parchment".
– Alopecia of affected areas is usually cicatricial (scarring) and permanent.
– Sunlight may exacerbate lesions.
– Systemic involvement is rare, but fever, weight loss, proteinuria, haemolytic anaemia, thrombocytopenia, and arthropathy may be encountered.

Diagnosis
• Histopathological examination and immunofluorescence or immunohistochemistry of biopsies of affected skin:
– Changes are centred on the dermo-epidermal junction, consisting of an interface dermatitis which may be hydropic (cell-poor) or lichenoid (cell-rich) or mixed, with focal thickening of the basement membrane zone and pigmentary incontinence.
– Immunoglobulin (IgG) and, or, complement may be demonstrated as a linear band (lupus band) at the basement membrane zone.
• Cases with systemic signs should have samples submitted for routine haematology, biochemistry panels, and urinalysis to detect other

organ involvement, followed by additional immunological tests such as the antinuclear antibody (ANA) test and Coombs test. A positive ANA titre is seen in most cases with systemic involvement.
- Differentials to be considered may be numerous, and include idiopathic leucoderma (vitiligo), pemphigus foliaceus, generalised or localised granulomatous disease (sarcoidosis), multisystemic eosinophilic epitheliotropic disease, vasculitis, erythema multiforme, adverse drug reaction, idiopathic seborrhoea, and epitheliotropic lymphoma.

Treatment
- CLE without systemic involvement can be managed by use of topical anti-inflammatory drugs and sunlight avoidance. Prognosis is usually good, but treatment usually needs to be continued for life:
  - Hydrocortisone in the form of hydrocortisone aceponate spray (Cortavance Spray, Virbac) marketed for small animals, applied once daily initially then 2–3 times weekly to maintain remission; alternatively, over-the-counter human hydrocortisone 1% cream.
  - More potent steroids such as triamcinolone and betamethasone can be used, in the form of products licensed for use in small animals (e.g. Dermanolon spray, Dechra, containing triamcinolone and salicylic acid) or for humans, often in conjunction with an antibiotic.
  - Off-label use of tacrolimus (Protopic 0.1% Ointment, Leo Pharma) avoids potential steroid-related side effects of skin thinning and inhibition of hair growth; daily application until inflammation is controlled, then 2–3 times weekly as needed to control the condition.
- Severe or extensive cases may require systemic corticosteroids to achieve remission, e.g. prednisolone 1–2 mg/kg every 24 hours; once in remission topical therapy is used for maintenance.
- Avoidance of sunlight is indicated, may control mild cases, and benefits all cases as depigmented areas are prone to sunburn. House from 8 a.m. to 5 p.m. and use of topical sunscreens.
- Cases with systemic involvement require immunosuppressive therapy as outlined for pemphigus foliaceus; response to therapy is unpredictable. Prognosis is better with earlier diagnosis and initiation of therapy.

Immune-mediated vasculitis

Most cases of vasculitis present with ulcerated lesions (see Chapter 4) but crusting can be the predominant presenting sign.

Pastern leucocytoclastic vasculitis

Clinical features
- A specific clinico-pathological entity recognised in horses of either sex, affecting non-pigmented lower limbs, and most often reported in summer months.
- Aetiopathogenesis is poorly understood, but most cases have a history of previous episodes of chronic or recurrent pastern dermatitis, and an association with both staphylococcal infection and *Pseudomonas* infection has been reported. Immune-complex deposits (IgG and, or, complement) have been identified in the blood vessel walls, suggestive of a type III hypersensitivity. Involvement of non-pigmented skin may reflect the deleterious effects of ultraviolet light on skin immune function and increased risk of infection as predisposing factors.
- Signs:
  - Usually restricted to non-pigmented lower limbs and may affect only one or multiple limbs. Occasionally extends to pigmented skin.
  - Lesions, which affect medial, lateral, and sometimes palmar/plantar aspects of pastern, fetlock, and distal metacarpal/metatarsal regions, are usually multiple to coalescing and well demarcated (Figure 3.16).

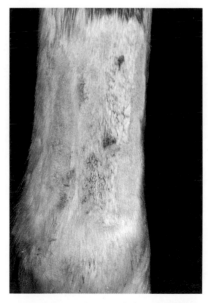

Figure 3.16 Leucocytoclastic vasculitis. Tightly adherent crusts overlying haemorrhagic, ulcerated lesions of the metatarsal region.

- Initially erythema, ulceration, oozing, and crusting are seen, sometimes with marked oedema.
- Chronically, lesions acquire a rough, warty surface which is tightly adherent to the underlying skin and difficult to remove.
- Lesions are painful.

Diagnosis
- History, signs – lesions confined to distal, non-pigmented skin of limbs.
- Histopathology:
  - Changes primarily involve the small blood vessels in the superficial dermis.
  - Leucocytoclastic vasculitis, vessel wall necrosis, and thrombosis are seen acutely, and vessel wall thickening and hyalinisation are chronic changes.
  - A mixed perivascular infiltrate is found in the dermis.
  - Overlying epidermal changes include hyperplasia with rete peg formation and variable hydropic degeneration.
- Differentials: rule out bacterial pyoderma as differential or ongoing predisposing factor; other major differential is photosensitisation, particularly contact type; differentiate clinically and by liver function tests.

Treatment
- Address any pre-existing or co-existing bacterial infection with appropriate systemic antibiosis as described earlier.
- Topical therapy with soaks and keratoplastic agents to remove crusts and debris; sedation may be needed.
- Systemic corticosteroids in high anti-inflammatory to immunosuppressive doses where vasculitis is confirmed:
  - Prednisolone 1–2 mg/kg once daily by mouth for the first 2 weeks with gradual tapering to alternate-day dosing and withdrawal over following 2–4 weeks.
- Occasionally, recurrence of lesions after withdrawal of steroids requires a further course of therapy.

Drug eruptions

See Chapter 4.

ENVIRONMENTAL CAUSES

Contact dermatitis

Clinical features
- May involve irritant and, or, hypersensitivity mechanisms.
- Localised lesions at contact sites, promoted by moisture (sweating), and can affect both haired and hairless areas.
- Causes may include:
  - Mechanical abrasion of the skin due to ill-fitting or poorly maintained tack, or working the horse on a muddy or gritty terrain.
  - Chemical contact dermatitis most commonly follows the inappropriate application of skin medicaments, or exposure to stable disinfectants and cleaning agents used on harness or rugs.
  - Allergic sensitisers include dyes and preservatives, soaps, topical medicaments, plants, forage, chemicals.
  - Caustic or corrosive chemicals (Figure 3.17).
- Signs:
  - Severity is dependent upon the nature of the irritant involved, but a low-grade inflammation accompanied by scaling and hair loss is common (Figure 3.18).
  - Variable pruritus may be present.
  - More severe reactions present with oedema, blistering, hair loss, exfoliation, and weeping erosions or ulcerations.

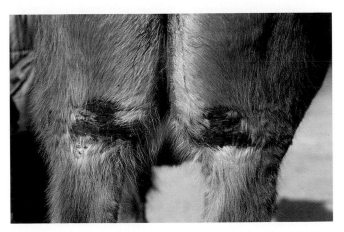

Figure 3.17 Irritant contact dermatitis caused by leaning against a fence coated with creosote.

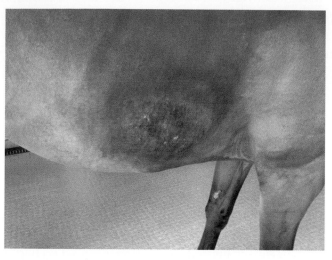

Figure 3.18 Contact dermatitis. Circumscribed patch of scaling, alopecia, and hyperpigmentation, bilaterally symmetrical, on lateral trunk associated with leather dressing used on rider's boots.

Diagnosis
- Lesions are confined to the contact areas, and together with the history, usually give an indication as to the nature of the causative agent.
- Histopathological changes are non-specific, with a neutrophilic to mixed superficial perivascular dermal infiltrate and variable epithelial changes from acanthosis to spongiosis and ulceration.
- Patch testing can be considered, but is often not practicable.

Treatment
- Prevent further exposure to the agent.
- Remove the agent from the skin surface by washing.
- Symptomatic palliative therapy as required (anti-inflammatory drugs, topical or systemic glucocorticoids; protective dressings; control of secondary infection).

Toxicoses

Crusting and scaling are common signs in several chemical toxicoses. Hair loss is also commonly seen, and may be more prominent than scaling – see Chapter 6 (arsenic, mercury, and selenium toxicoses).

Iodism

Clinical features
- Iodine toxicosis usually follows excessive administration of iodides in the treatment of cutaneous mycoses, although this is now considered to be a substandard method of treating fungal diseases in horses. Signs are generalised dryness and scaling of the skin with variable alopecia and watering of the eyes and nose.

Diagnosis
- History of iodide administration, clinical signs.

Treatment
- Iodine is rapidly metabolised and excreted and once the source of iodine is removed, the condition resolves.

UNCERTAIN AETIOLOGY

Hyperaesthetic leucotrichia

Clinical features
- Rare dermatosis of uncertain aetiology reported in the USA. May be an unusual form of erythema multiforme (see Chapter 5) as some cases have been associated with herpesvirus infection or rhinopneumonitis vaccination.
- No age, breed, or sex predisposition.
- Signs:
  - Lesions may be single or multiple, and are found on the dorsal midline between the withers and the tail base.
  - Early lesions consist of focal crusts 1–5 mm in diameter.
  - There is a marked degree of pain associated with this condition, which may precede the development of crusts.
  - Within a few weeks white hairs appear at the site of the lesions, the pain subsides; crusts disappear over a period of 1–3 months, but the leucotrichia is permanent.

Diagnosis
- Clinical appearance is usually distinctive. Confirm with histopathology, which characteristically shows hydropic interface dermatitis with apoptosis of keratinocytes, satellitosis of lymphocytes and macrophages, pigmentary incontinence, and variable dermal oedema in addition to surface crusting.

Treatment

- Corticosteroids, even at high doses, are of only limited value. The disease usually runs its own course.

Generalised granulomatous disease (Sarcoidosis)

Clinical features

- Characterised by generalised granuloma formation in skin and internal organs; appears to be analogous to human sarcoidosis (not to be confused with equine sarcoids).
- Aetiology unknown but presumed to be an abnormal host response to as yet unidentified antigens. The role of the plant, hairy vetch, and relevance of positive *Borrelia burgdorferi* antibody titres are uncertain. Mycobacterial infection implicated in one case although PCR findings were negative in other reports.
- Signs:
  - Skin involvement in most cases.
  - Cutaneous lesions most commonly consist of scaling and crusting with variable alopecia, which may be focal, multifocal, or generalised (Figures 3.19 and 3.20).
  - Nodular lesions are less common, but may co-exist with the scaling lesions.
  - Systemic signs include weight loss and decreased appetite, and a persistent low-grade fever is common.
  - Internal organ involvement may include the lungs, lymph nodes, liver, gastrointestinal tract, spleen, kidney, bones, and central nervous system.

Diagnosis

- Laboratory findings:
  - May include leucocytosis, mild anaemia, elevated fibrinogen, hyperglobulinaemia, and abnormal hepatic and renal function.
- Histopathology:
  - Diagnosis is confirmed by identification of typical non-caseating granulomas comprised of epithelioid and multinucleate histiocytic giant cells. These are found in all organs involved.
  - Biopsies of skin and peripheral lymph nodes of greatest value.
  - No aetiological agents found on special staining.
- Differentials include dermatophilosis, dermatophytosis, pemphigus foliaceus, cutaneous adverse drug reaction, contact dermatitis, generalised seborrhoea, CLE, epitheliotropic lymphoma, toxicoses.

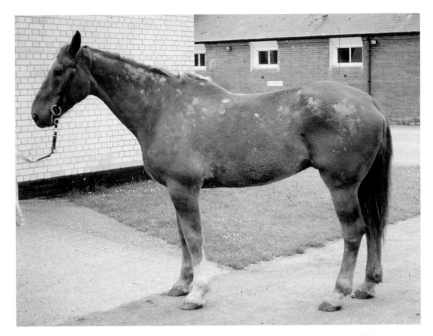

Figure 3.19 Generalised patchy alopecia and scaling in a 9-year-old hunter with generalised granulomatous disease. Note poor bodily condition. Lymphadenopathy was also present.

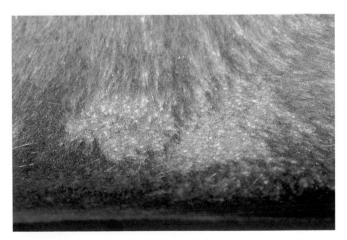

Figure 3.20 Cutaneous lesions of scaling and alopecia in generalised granulomatous disease.

Treatment

- Most cases respond well to glucocorticoid therapy at high anti-inflammatory to immunosuppressive doses (prednisolone 1.5–4 mg/kg once daily) with tapering to alternate-day therapy as lesions improve.

- Prognosis is less good if signs of internal involvement and wasting are present.
- Some cases may go into prolonged remission, others suffer relapses which require further treatment, and some need continuing treatment to maintain remission.

Localised sarcoidosis

Clinical features
- Isolated, hyperkeratotic, crusted, alopecic plaques occur particularly on the limbs (Figure 3.21), occasionally elsewhere.
- Distal limb lesions are occasionally associated with lameness.
- Affected animals are typically otherwise healthy, with no systemic signs or internal organ involvement.

Diagnosis
- Clinical signs, histopathological confirmation of sarcoidal granulomatous dermatitis as above.

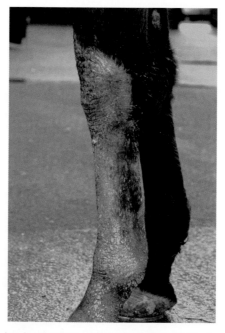

Figure 3.21 Localised sarcoidosis. Alopecia, scaling, lichenification, and thickening of the distal limb in an aged thoroughbred mare.

Treatment
- Early, small lesions may respond to topical glucocorticoids, but an initial course of systemic steroids as above is usually needed.
- Response to treatment is variable, and in cases where remission is achieved continuing maintenance therapy is usually needed.

Multisystemic eosinophilic epitheliotropic disease (MEED)

Clinical features
- Rare sporadic condition characterised by tissue eosinophilia affecting the skin, oral cavity, salivary glands, gastrointestinal tract, pancreas, biliary epithelium, and bronchial epithelium. The aetiology is unknown.
- Generally affects young animals; Standardbreds and Thoroughbreds are predisposed.
- Signs:
  - Skin lesions characterised by exudation, scaling, and crusting with alopecia (Figure 3.22) and areas of ulceration (Figure 3.23).
  - Coronary band, face, and oral mucosa are affected initially with progression to a generalised exfoliative dermatitis.
  - Intense pruritus with self-mutilation is present in some horses.
  - Chronic weight loss is common, often without loss of appetite. Passing of loose faeces is seen in about 50% of cases and dependent oedema is commonly present.

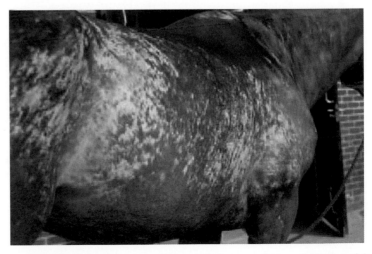

Figure 3.22 Multisystemic eosinophilic epitheliotropic disease (MEED): exfoliation, excoriation, and alopecia on the trunk.

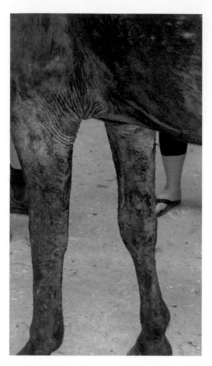

Figure 3.23 Alopecia, scaling, and areas of ulceration affecting the forelimbs of a horse with MEED. Source: Courtesy of Greg Burton.

- Affected horses are usually dull and lethargic and may be febrile.
- Thickened bowel wall, thickened mesentery, and enlarged lymph nodes may be detected on rectal examination.

Diagnosis
- Biopsies of skin show:
  - Mixed inflammatory reaction patterns with eosinophils predominating, together with lymphocytes and plasma cells.
  - Marked and irregular epidermal hyperplasia with mixed orthokeratotic and parakeratotic hyperkeratosis.
  - Epitheliotropic infiltration of eosinophils and lymphocytes with apoptotic keratinocytes.
  - Eosinophilic microabscesses, eosinophilic folliculitis, and furunculosis may be seen.
- Rectal biopsies show similar eosinophilic inflammatory infiltrate.
- Low total plasma protein and albumin concentrations, reduced carbohydrate absorption.

- Differentials: pemphigus foliaceus, CLE, generalised granulomatous disease, bullous pemphigoid, pemphigus vulgaris, vasculitis, hepatocutaneous syndrome, erythema multiforme, epitheliotropic lymphoma, cutaneous drug reactions, toxicoses.

Treatment
- Prognosis is poor; most cases suffer progressive dermatitis and wasting resulting in death.
- Glucocorticoids at immunosuppressive doses may give some amelioration if given early in the disease; cases that respond require continuing treatment. Horses with the wasting syndrome do not usually respond.

Linear keratosis and alopecia

Clinical features
- A rare, distinctive dermatosis of unknown cause, seen most commonly in Quarterhorses, Standardbreds, and Thoroughbreds; usually seen in young animals.
- Lesions consist of asymptomatic, unilateral, vertical, linear band(s), variable crusting and scaling, coalescing papules, and alopecia, predominantly affecting the neck and thorax. Lesions may also occur on legs (Figure 3.24), hip, and pectoral regions.

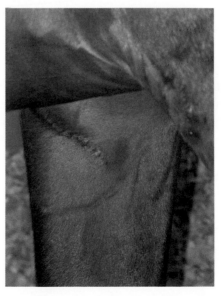

Figure 3.24 Linear keratosis. Line of crusted papules affecting medial aspect of upper forelimb, running from medial aspect of elbow in a cranio-distal direction.

Diagnosis
- Characteristic appearance. Histologically, there is papillated epidermal hyperplasia and marked hyperkeratosis with a mild superficial perivascular lymphocytic dermatitis. Lymphocytic to lymphohistiocytic mural folliculitis with destruction of the follicle is seen in cases of linear alopecia. It is uncertain if the alopecic form is a variant of the same disease as linear keratosis or a distinct entity.

Treatment
- Symptomatic treatment with keratolytic/keratoplastic shampoos or lotion (e.g. small animal shampoos: Coatex Medicated Shampoo, Vet Plus; Malabeze, Forte Healthcare; Sebomild, Virbac; Zincoseb Shampoo or Spray, Vetruus; Johnsons Skin Calm Shampoo; human selenium sulphide shampoo: Selsun; Dermisol Cream or Lotion, Zoetis UK) and topical glucocorticoids or tacrolimus may result in temporary improvement, but lesions do not fully resolve.

Cannon keratosis

Clinical features
- Rare, distinctive condition affecting cranial aspect of metatarsal regions and occasionally cranial metacarpal regions of middle aged to older horses, with no breed or sex predilection. Unknown aetiopathology; earlier theory of urine splatter causing lesions in stallions ("stud crud") is no longer credible.

Diagnosis
- Circumscribed papules and plaques of scaling and crusting with variable alopecia, without pruritus or inflammation, affecting the cranial aspect of both hind cannon bone and occasionally front cannon bone regions.
- Lesions can become fissured, inflamed, and secondarily infected.
- Usually a lifelong affliction.
- Histological findings include moderate to marked epidermal hyperplasia with marked hyperkeratosis, with mild mixed superficial perivascular dermatitis.

Treatment
- Symptomatic control with regular applications of topical keratolytic/keratoplastic shampoos, creams, lotions with or without antimicrobial activity (e.g. small animal shampoos: Coatex Medicated

Shampoo, Vet Plus; Malabeze, Forte Healthcare; Sebomild, Virbac; Zincoseb Shampoo or Spray, Vetruus; Johnsons Skin Calm Shampoo; human selenium sulphide shampoo: Selsun Blue, Sanofi; Dermisol Cream or Lotion, Zoetis UK).
- Topical glucocorticoids may be helpful in severe cases.

Coronary band dystrophy

Clinical features
- An uncommon, idiopathic, acquired keratinisation disorder affecting the coronary band of mature horses, particularly large or heavy breeds.
- This is a diagnosis of exclusion, made after eliminating other possible causes of coronitis.
- Signs:
  - All or part of coronary bands of all feet affected.
  - Lesions of proliferative hyperkeratosis of coronary band tissue (Figure 3.25) with variable fissuring, exudation, and crusting. Associated hoof wall changes may be seen in chronic cases. Ergots and chestnuts may be affected.
  - Severe cases may show lameness.

Diagnosis
- Histological examination of multiple tangential shave biopsies of coronary band tissue after abaxial sesamoid nerve blocks; samples taken with a large scalpel blade over the curvature of the heel, from haired skin through to the horny tissue are associated with low risk of future hoof wall defects. Samples should be deep enough to

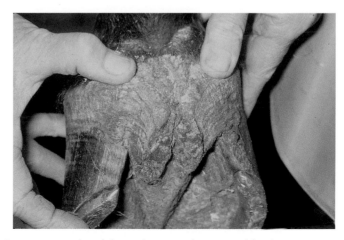

Figure 3.25 Coronary band dystrophy in a Belgian warmblood.

include basement membrane zone and some superficial dermis. Haemostasis is achieved by whole foot bandaging.

- Changes described include epidermal papillary hyperplasia with papillary squirting (spongiosis) over tips of dermal papillae, with overlying hyperkeratosis, which may be parakeratotic.
- Must rule out other causes of coronitis, in particular pemphigus foliaceus in mature horses, which often involves hoof, ergots, and chestnuts and may need multiple biopsies to capture the classical intraepithelial vesicopustules with acantholytic cells.
- Other differentials include:
  - Infection/infestation of the coronary band: chorioptic mange, dermatophilosis, staphylococcal pastern folliculitis, dermatophytosis.
  - Hepatocutaneous syndrome (superficial necrolytic dermatitis): exudative and ulcerative coronitis, associated weight loss, abnormal liver function tests.
  - Eosinophilic exfoliative dermatitis as part of MEED: exudative and ulcerative coronitis, associated with chronic eosinophilic enteritis, weight loss, diarrhoea.
  - Selenium toxicosis: coronary band separation with associated loss of mane and tail hair.
  - Seborrhoea: in severe generalised disease, there may be coronary band involvement.
  - Neoplasia: sarcoid, keratoma.

Treatment
- Symptomatic and palliative.
- Prognosis for improvement appears poor.

Greasy heel syndrome (Scratches, Cracked Heels)

Clinical features
- A variety of inflammatory skin conditions may affect the lower limb and pastern regions of the horse, and a number of terms may be used to describe the syndrome, including grease or greasy heels, cracked heels, scratches, and mud fever.
- None of these terms refers to a specific disease entity. They describe a clinical presentation that is common to a number of diseases (see Table 3.1).
- Signs:
  - Non-pigmented extremities are often involved.
  - Initial lesions affect the palmar or plantar aspect of the pastern region, but may extend laterally, medially, and proximally.

Table 3.1 Diseases to be considered as underlying causes of greasy heel syndrome.

Bacterial infections		
	Bacterial folliculitis/furunculosis	*Staphylococcus aureus*
		Beta-haemolytic *streptococci*
		Corynebacterium spp.
		Gram-negative bacilli
		Anaerobes
	Dermatophilosis	*Dermatophilus congolensis*
Fungal infections		
	Dermatophytosis	*Trichophyton equinum*
		T. mentagrophytes
		T. verrucosum
		Microsporum equinum
		M. gypseum
	Yeast infections	*Malassezia* dermatitis
		Candidiasis
Parasitic infestations		See Chapter 2
	Chorioptic mange	*Chorioptes bovis*
	Trombiculidiasis	*Neotrombicula autumnalis* larvae
	Pediculosis	*Bovicola equi*
		Haematopinus asini
Environmental causes		
	Trauma, over-reaches	See Chapter 4
	Contact dermatitis	
	Primary photosensitivity	See Chapter 4
Immune-mediated diseases		
	Pemphigus foliaceous	
	Leucocytoclastic vasculitis	
	Cutaneous lupus erythematosus	
Neoplasia		See Chapter 5
	Sarcoid	
	Squamous cell carcinoma	
	Keratoma	
Nutritional/metabolic		
	Secondary (hepatic) photosensitisation	
	Hepatocutaneous syndrome	See Chapter 4
	Chronic selenosis	See Chapter 6
Uncertain aetiology		
	Localised/generalised granulomatous disease	
	Eosinophilic exfoliative dermatitis (MEED)	
	Generalised seborrhoea	
	Coronary band dystrophy	
	Chronic proliferative pododermatitis (canker)	See Chapter 5
	Idiopathic pastern dermatitis	
	Chronic progressive lymphoedema	See Chapter 5

- Erythema, oozing, and hair loss are common early signs progressing to crust formation (Figure 3.26 and Figure 3.27).
- Ulceration may occur, particularly if there is underlying vasculitis.
- Chronically thickening of the skin with fissuring develops.

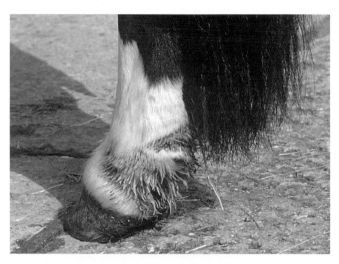

Figure 3.26   Exudative pastern dermatitis – 'greasy heels'.

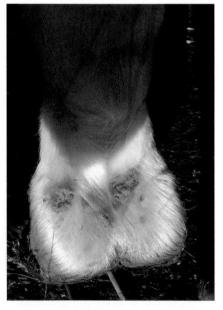

Figure 3.27   Focal crusting regions in a case of chronic pastern dermatitis – 'scratches'.

Diagnosis
- It is important that underlying causes be identified so that proper therapeutic measures can be instigated.
- Superficial adhesive tape samples, crusts, and scrapes should be examined for *Chorioptes* mites, *Dermatophilus* organisms, and fungal elements, and samples submitted for bacterial and fungal culture.
- Liver enzymes and bile acids should be evaluated if lesions are restricted to non-pigmented skin to rule out secondary photosensitisation.
- Skin biopsies may be indicated for conventional histopathology, tissue culture, and immunofluorescence/immunohistochemistry.

Treatment
- Depends upon the cause, but should include:
  - Removal of crusts (see section on dermatophilosis) and thorough cleansing, prevention of further damage by irritants, moisture, and sunlight. Ensure adequate contact time with antibacterial/antifungal shampoos, thoroughly dry after rinsing. Irritant or astringent compounds should be avoided.
  - Topical anti-inflammatory preparations with antibacterial and antifungal activity are frequently used.
  - Stable horse on clean, dry, soft bedding.
  - If vasculitis is identified then high-dose systemic corticosteroid therapy is indicated, alongside attention to predisposing or concurrent infectious agents.
- In idiopathic cases, routine cleansing on a prophylactic basis and protection of affected areas (e.g. stable boots and pastern boots lined with a layer of activated carbon cloth impregnated with a microscopic nano silver; Equi-Med AG) with judicious use of corticosteroids may be the best approach.

REFERENCES AND FURTHER READING

BEVA resources for vets Protect ME antimicrobial policy guidance, www.beva.org.uk//Portals/0/Documents/ResourcesForVets/1beva-antimicrobial-policy-template-distributed.pdf

Figueredo, L.A., Cafarchia, C., and Otranto, D. (2011) *Geotrichum candidum* as etiological agent of horse dermatomycosis. *Veterinary Microbiology*, 148: 368–371.

Islam, M.Z., Espinosa-Gongora, C., Damborg, P. et al. (2017) Horses in Denmark are a reservoir of diverse clones of methicillin-resistant and -susceptible *Staphylococcus aureus*. *Frontiers in Microbiology*, 8: 543.

Lloyd, D.H. and Page, S.W. (2018) Antimicrobial stewardship in veterinary medicine. *Microbiology Spectrum*, 6 (3). doi: 10.1128/microbiolspec.ARBA-0023-2017.

Panzuti, P., Rocafort Ferrer, G., Mosca, M. et al. (2020) Equine pastern vasculitis in a horse associated with a multidrug-resistant *Pseudomonas aeruginosa* isolate. *Veterinary Dermatology*, 31: 247–e55.

Raidal, S.L. (2019) Antimicrobial stewardship in equine practice. *Australian Veterinary Journal*, 97: 238–242.

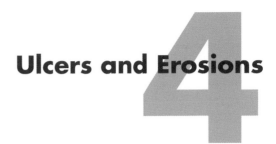

Ulcers and Erosions 4

CONTAGIOUS CAUSES

Helminth infestation

Cutaneous habronemiasis (summer sores)

Clinical features
- Cutaneous lesions caused by the larvae of one of three *Habronema* spp. (*H. muscae*, *H. microstoma*, *H. (Draschia) megastoma*); adults live in the stomach of equidae; eggs and larvae in faeces are ingested by flies acting as intermediate hosts (*Musca domestica*, the house fly, and *Stomoxys calcitrans*, the stable fly), infective larvae are deposited on the horse in moist areas such as mucocutaneous regions and wounds. Larvae deposited around the lips are swallowed and complete the life cycle.
- Skin lesions result from aberrant parasitism when larvae are deposited on moist or damaged skin.
- Hypersensitivity is believed to be involved in aetiopathogenesis of lesions.
- Prevalence has reduced with widespread use of avermectins, more common in warmer climates but now rare in the UK.
- Signs:
  - Ulcerated papules and nodules around eyes, of conjunctivae, periorally (Figure 4.1), and of external genitalia and distal extremities.
  - Seen in summer months, often only affecting individual horses in a group.

Practical Equine Dermatology, Second Edition. Janet D. Littlewood, David H. Lloyd and J. Mark Craig.
© 2022 John Wiley & Sons Ltd. Published 2022 by John Wiley & Sons Ltd.

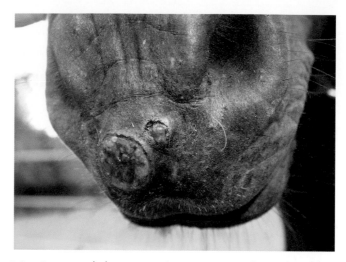

Figure 4.1 Cutaneous habronemiasis (summer sores): ulcerated nodular lesions on the muzzle. Source: Courtesy of Kieran O'Brien.

   – May complicate lesions of exuberant granulation tissue and ulcerated tumours.

Diagnosis
- Clinical signs, seasonal occurrence, worming history.
- Occasionally larvae are seen in smears from lesions; chance of detection is increased by microscopical examination of sediment following centrifugation of scrapings suspended in saline.
- Biopsy reveals nodular to diffuse eosinophilic dermatitis with discrete areas of coagulation necrosis, where nematode larvae are found.
- Differentials include exuberant granulation tissue, eosinophilic granuloma, sarcoid, squamous cell carcinoma, bacterial and fungal granuloma.

Treatment
- Ivermectin (Bimectin Horse Oral Paste, Bimeda; Animec Oral Paste for Horses, Chanelle Pharma; Eqvalan Oral Paste for Horses, Boehringer Ingelheim Animal Health UK; Vectin Horse Oral Paste, MSD Animal Health UK; Eraquell Oral Paste, Virbac; Noromectin, Norbrook Laboratories) 200 µg/kg or moxidectin (Equest Oral Gel for Horses and Ponies, Zoetis UK) 400 µg/kg, two doses given by mouth at 3-week interval kills larvae, and lesions usually resolve promptly.
- Systemic glucocorticoids reportedly effective as sole treatment, but in conjunction with avermectin therapy secure rapid response with resolution of most lesions in 7–14 days.

- Topical preparations containing steroids applied under bandages can be effective for lesions on the limbs.
- Lesions that fail to resolve or involve exuberant granulation tissue may require surgical debridement and dressings.
- Prophylaxis consists of inclusion of avermectins in deworming programmes and fly control.

Parafilariasis

Clinical features
- Adult *Parafilaria multipapillosa* worms are found in nodules in subcutaneous and intermuscular connective tissues; these nodules ulcerate and discharge a haemorrhagic exudate containing eggs and larvae with various flies serving as vectors or intermediate hosts.
- Disease has summer incidence; cases are reported in Great Britain and Europe.
- Papules and nodules appear suddenly over the neck, shoulders, and trunk, usually non-painful, which open to the surface; bloody exudate dries to reddish-black crusts, followed by healing.
- New lesions continue to occur as older lesions heal.
- Spontaneous resolution in autumn and winter.
- Many cases recur annually for 3–4 years and then spontaneously resolve.

Diagnosis
- Direct smears reveal presence of larvae, embryonated eggs, and numerous eosinophils.
- Biopsies show nodular to diffuse eosinophilic dermatitis with coiled adult nematodes surrounded by necrotic debris.
- Differentials include bacterial, fungal, and parasitic granulomas and hypodermiasis.

Treatment
- Avermectins (ivermectin (Bimectin Horse Oral Paste, Bimeda; Animec Oral Paste for Horses, Chanelle Pharma; Eqvalan Oral Paste for Horses, Boehringer Ingelheim Animal Health UK; Vectin Horse Oral Paste, MSD Animal Health UK; Eraquell Oral Paste, Virbac; Noromectin, Norbrook Laboratories) 200 µg/kg or moxidectin (Equest Oral Gel for Horses and Ponies, Zoetis UK) 400 µg/kg,), two oral doses at 3-week intervals should secure resolution of lesions.

Viral infections

Coital exanthema

Clinical features
- Caused by equine herpesvirus (EHV)-3, the disease is spread by coitus, fomites, and insect vectors.
- Signs:
  - Incubation period of 5–9 days before development of lesions consisting of papules and vesicles, which ulcerate, and crusts affecting the penis, prepuce, and scrotum of stallions (Figure 4.2) and the vulva and perineum of mares (Figure 4.3).
  - Lips, mouth, and nostrils may also be involved.
  - Healing is usually complete in 14 days, although focal depigmentation (see Chapter 7) may persist. Secondary infection may complicate the primary lesions.
  - High percentage of horses become latent carriers, with recrudescence of disease and clinical signs in association with onset of breeding season; systemic glucocorticoids and other stresses may also cause reactivation of disease.

Diagnosis
- Coital exanthema must be differentiated from other viral infections and immune-mediated conditions such as bullous pemphigoid and other genital infections.
- Biopsy specimens reveal ballooning degeneration of basal epithelium and vesicle formation. Intranuclear inclusion bodies may be identified.

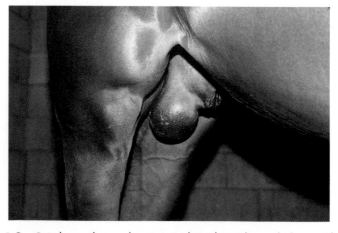

Figure 4.2 Coital exanthema showing epidermal vesicles and ulcers with marked scrotal swelling.

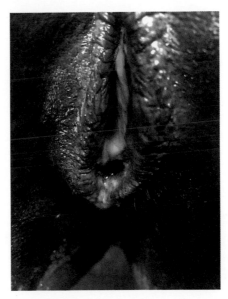

Figure 4.3   Vulval lesions of EHV-3 infection. Source: Courtesy of Sarah Moore.

- Diagnosis can be confirmed by virus isolation from vesicle contents, crusts or biopsy samples, identification of virus in samples by electron microscopy, or demonstration of a rising antibody titre to EHV-3. PCR-identification of EHV-3 in skin lesions is available from some laboratories.
- No test currently available to detect latent carriers of EHV-3.

Treatment
- Control of secondary infection with topical antiseptic washes and emollients; systemic antibiotics may be necessary in severe cases.
- Stud animals should be rested from mating, including teasing, for 3–4 weeks.
- Disinfection of potential fomites including grooming equipment and sponges.

Equine herpesvirus-1 dermatitis

Clinical features
- Rarely, EHV-1 rhinopneumonitis may be accompanied by ulcerative mucocutaneous lesions.
- Signs:
  - Ulcers and crusted papules affecting periorbital and perioral regions, muzzle, nostrils, oral mucosa, other mucocutaneous junctions, and skin.

– Concurrent signs of EHV-1 infection – cough, fever, oculonasal discharge, lymphadenopathy.

Diagnosis
- Clinical signs.
- Histopathology; intranuclear viral inclusion bodies in cells of epidermis and adnexa.
- Confirmation by virus isolation or PCR.
- Differentials include other viral dermatitides (EHV-3 dermatitis, vesicular stomatitis), bacterial pyoderma, vasculitis, drug eruption, erythema multiforme, pemphigus vulgaris, systemic lupus erythematosus.

Treatment
- Supportive therapy including systemic antibiotics to address secondary bacterial bronchopneumonia.
- Isolation to limit spread of infection, disinfection of potential fomites.

Horse pox

Clinical features
- A now rare, benign disease of horses. The aetiological agent is an orthopoxvirus related to, but distinct from, vaccinia virus.
- Signs:
  - Three clinical presentations are described:
    - Oral lesions.
    - Pastern and fetlock lesions.
    - Vulval lesions.
  - Vesicles, umbilicated pustules, and crusts affecting the skin and mucosal surfaces.
  - Mild pyrexia may occur.
  - Horses with limb involvement may be lame.

Diagnosis
- Ballooning degeneration of epidermal cells is seen on biopsy, with intraepidermal vesicles and intracytoplasmic inclusion bodies.
- Demonstration of poxvirus by electron microscopy and virus isolation confirms the diagnosis.

Treatment
- The natural course of the disease is 2–4 weeks and recovered horses have long-term immunity.

Vesicular stomatitis

Clinical features
- A notifiable disease of livestock, including horses, not reported to date in the UK, but enzootic in the Americas; caused by a lyssavirus of the *Rhabdoviridae* family, transmitted by flies and contact with infected secretions and aerosols.
- Signs:
  - Excessive salivation in association with vesicles, which progress to painful ulcers, on the lips, tongue, and oral cavity; occasionally oedema of the head develops.
  - Ulcerated blisters of the coronary band with accompanying lameness; may progress to severe hoof wall defects and even sloughing of the hoof.
  - Lesions may also be seen in genital and mammary areas.
  - Lethargy, malaise, and fever.
  - Post-inflammatory depigmentation.

Diagnosis
- Suspected cases must be reported immediately to relevant government animal health authorities.
- Confirmation of diagnosis by virus isolation and rising serum antibody titres.

Treatment
- No specific treatment, healing usually occurs within 2 weeks.
- Management of outbreaks in accordance with guidance from state veterinary services, with appropriate biosecurity and quarantine procedures.

IMMUNE-MEDIATED CAUSES

Pemphigus vulgaris

Clinical features
- Extremely rare autoimmune disease in the horse associated with auto-antibodies against the epithelial desmosomal protein desmoglein 3.
- Vesicles and bullae progress to painful ulcers, affecting the mouth and upper gastrointestinal tract and mucocutaneous junctions.

Diagnosis
- Biopsies reveal suprabasilar clefts and vesicles with acantholytic keratinocytes.
- Intercellular deposits of immunoglobulin can be demonstrated by immunofluorescent staining.
- Differentials include bullous pemphigoid, paraneoplastic pemphigus/pemphigoid, cutaneous lupus erythematosus, and viral diseases such as herpes coital exanthema and vesicular stomatitis.

Treatment
- Prognosis is grave, with minimal temporary response to immunosuppressive doses of corticosteroids; no effective treatment reported.

Bullous pemphigoid

Clinical features
- A very rare autoimmune disease resulting from auto-antibodies directed against antigens at the dermo-epidermal junction.
- Signs:
  - Primary lesions are vesicles or bullae that rapidly ulcerate, affecting skin, mucocutaneous junctions, and oral mucosa. The axillary and inguinal areas are particularly affected.
  - Ulcers, crusts, and epidermal collarettes are the usual signs, with pain; excessive salivation is seen if oral involvement is significant.
  - Affected animals are severely unwell, with anorexia, fever, and depression.

Diagnosis
- Biopsy findings of subepidermal vesicular dermatitis are strongly suggestive.
- Direct immunofluorescence or immunohistochemistry may demonstrate linear deposits of immunoglobulin and, usually, complement at the dermo-epidermal junction, in the absence of previous steroid therapy.
- Differentials include viral diseases such as herpes coital exanthema, horse pox and vesicular stomatitis, pemphigus vulgaris, paraneoplastic pemphigus/pemphigoid, cutaneous lupus erythematosus, erythema multiforme, and drug eruptions.

Treatment
- The prognosis is grave with poor response to immunosuppressive doses of steroids.

Paraneoplastic pemphigus/pemphigoid

Rare cases of horses with ulcerated oral lesions, characterised by supra-basal epidermal bullae or subepidermal bullae, have been reported where lesions resolved after surgical removal of neoplastic lesions.

Vasculitis

Cutaneous vasculitis is an uncommon condition in the horse. Most cases are thought to be immune-mediated. Mechanisms may involve type III hypersensitivity where antigen-antibody complexes are deposited in the walls of blood vessels, and, or, secondary immune-mediated responses resulting from neutrophil-induced damage to endothelial cells. Vasculitis may be associated with infections, drug administration, systemic disease, neoplasia, and connective tissue disorders or may be idiopathic. The skin is primarily involved, but other organ systems may also be involved.

Purpura haemorrhagica

Clinical features
- Most common manifestation of cutaneous vasculitis, occurring after infection, or occasionally vaccination; most frequently follows strangles, caused by *Streptococcus equi*.
- Acute onset, usually 2–3 weeks post infection, variable severity and clinical course.
- Signs:
  - Oedema of face, distal limbs, ventrum, with heat and pain.
  - Petechiation and ecchymoses of mucosae.
  - In severe cases oozing, necrosis, ulceration, and sloughing.
  - Systemic signs of anorexia, depression, reluctance to move, but often without fever.
- Differentials include vasculitis due to other causes, severe urticaria, erythema multiforme, bullous pemphigoid, pemphigus vulgaris, adverse drug reactions.

Diagnosis
- History, clinical signs, known exposure to strangles cases.
- Classical histopathology in early lesions is neutrophilic vasculitis, fibrinoid necrosis of vessels, with segmental dermal necrosis; chronic lesions show hyalinised thickening of vessels, thrombosis, and occasional karyorrhectic nuclei.
- Positive antistreptococcal antibody titre to confirm.

- Rule out equine viral arteritis (notifiable disease) by serum neutralising antibody titres, equine infectious anaemia (notifiable disease) by Coggin's test and anaplasmosis (granulocytic ehrlichiosis) by looking for parasitic morulae in granulocytes, antibody titres, or PCR.

Treatment
- Identify and treat underlying cause.
- Immunosuppressive doses of glucocorticoids – prednisolone (2–4 mg/kg by mouth) once daily until in remission (7–21 days) then reduce to alternate-day dosing and gradually taper; alternatively oral dexamethasone may be given, but injections are best avoided in animals with a coagulopathy as serious bruising may occur.
- Concurrent azathioprine (2–3 mg/kg q 24 hours, off-label use) or pentoxifylline (10 mg/kg q 12 hours, off-label use) may be added in cases responding poorly to glucocorticoids.
- Antibiotic cover is usually indicated.
- Supportive therapy consisting of cold-water hosing, support bandages, walking in hand.
- Prognosis is generally good, unless animals are febrile.

Pastern leucocytoclastic vasculitis

See Chapter 3.

Erythema multiforme

Clinical features
- Uncommon, often self-limiting dermatosis occurring secondary to a number of preceding factors or diseases, the most common of which are:
  - Drugs (antimicrobials: potentiated sulphonamides, penicillins; ivermectin, topical, and non-medicinal chemicals).
  - Infections (viral, especially herpes, fungal, and bacterial).
  - Neoplasia, especially lymphoma.
  - Occasionally food triggers suspected.
- Many cases are idiopathic.
- Aetiology is poorly understood, thought to involve cell-mediated hypersensitivity response.
- Signs:
  - Acute, sometimes recurrent dermatosis, ranging in severity from mild to severe.
  - Lesions tend to be symmetrically distributed and mucous membranes may be involved.

- Clinical appearance can be wide-ranging, but usually consists of urticarial papules and plaques, vesicles and bullae, or a combination of both.
- Peripheral expansion and central resolution of lesions often result in annular, arciform, serpiginous, and polycyclic lesions, which must be differentiated from true or simple oedematous lesions of classical urticaria due to type 1 hypersensitivity reactions.
- As vesicles are short-lived, lesions are usually focal or multifocal erosions and ulcerations or crusts, at presentation.

Diagnosis

- A careful history is essential, noting previous drug administration and previous or concurrent illnesses.
- Histopathology:
  - Necrotic (apoptotic) keratinocytes in the epidermis and adnexal epithelium; lymphocytic exocytosis and satellitosis; vacuolar changes of the basal cell layer and, or, basement membrane zone; oedema of the superficial dermis; extravasated erythrocytes in the superficial dermis; superficial perivascular lymphohistiocytic infiltrate.
  - Subepidermal vesicle formation may arise due to vacuolar degeneration and, or, severe superficial dermal oedema.
  - Apoptosis of keratinocytes may be very extensive.
- Differentials: all diseases showing erosions or ulcers of the oral mucosa, mucocutaneous junctions, cutaneous vesicles or bullae, superficial erosions or ulcers, erythematous macules.

Treatment

- Mild cases undergo spontaneous resolution within weeks to months.
- Corticosteroids (prednisolone 1–2 mg/kg once daily by mouth, then reducing to alternate-day therapy when control is achieved) may be required in severe cases.

Cutaneous adverse drug reactions

Clinical features

- Reactions may occur to drugs or other chemicals gaining access to the body by any route, and may mimic virtually any dermatosis.
- Mechanisms involved are thought to be hypersensitivity reactions, but are poorly understood.

- Antibiotics, particularly potentiated sulphonamides and penicillins, are most commonly involved; other drugs that have been implicated include non-steroidal anti-inflammatory drugs, anaesthetic agents, ivermectin, vaccines, and multivitamins (Table 4.1) but, in theory, any drug could be involved.
- An adverse reaction may occur after the first exposure to a drug or after many years of use. Signs can appear with 24–48 hours of exposure, but commonly occur within 1–3 weeks, although may be delayed for as long as 2 months.
- Signs may mimic any skin disease, but certain features should lead to a high index of suspicion including:
  - Urticaria or angio-oedema (Figure 4.4).
  - Diffuse erythema.
  - Bilaterally symmetrical lesions.
  - Papular rashes (Figures 4.5 and 4.6).

Table 4.1   Cutaneous manifestations of adverse drug reactions

Frequency	Reaction pattern	Drugs implicated
Common	Urticaria / angio-oedema	Penicillin, tetracyclines, ciprofloxacin, streptomycin, sulphonamides, neomycin, phenylbutazone, flunixin, aspirin, acepromazine, guaifenesin, hormones, vaccines, antisera, vitamin B complex, iron dextrans, various topicals (shampoos, sprays, pour-ons, dips, gels)
	Exfoliative dermatitis – erythroderma	Trimethoprim-sulphonamides, various topicals (shampoos, sprays, pour-ons, dips)
	Erythema multiforme	Trimethoprim-sulphonamides, ceftiofur, vaccines
	Contact dermatitis	Various topical products and non-medical chemical contactants
Rare	Injection site panniculitis/vasculitis	Vaccines, other injectables
	Vasculitis	Trimethoprim-sulphonamides, penicillin, phenylbutazone, acepromazine, tiludronate
Very rare	Maculopapular	Phenylbutazone
	Pemphigus foliaceus	Penicillin
	Sterile pyogranuloma	Ivermectin
	Trichorrhexis and hypotrichosis	Ivermectin
	Tail head dermatitis	Moxidectin
	Epitheliotropic lymphoma-like	Drug combinations
	Intense pruritus	Morphine

Source: Scott and Miller (2011).

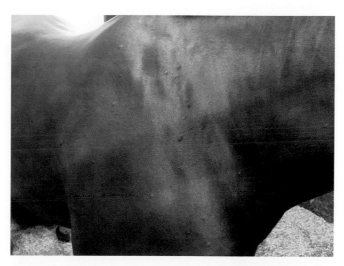

Figure 4.4 Urticarial wheals and plaques after application of car shampoo. Source: Courtesy of Kieran O'Brien.

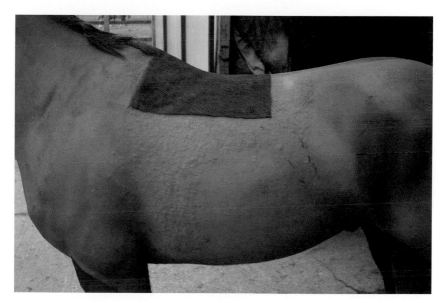

Figure 4.5 Maculopapular and urticarial eruptions after administration of trimethoprim-potentiated sulphonamides. Source: Courtesy of Kieran O'Brien.

- Sharply demarcated erosions and ulcerations.
- Vesicular and bullous eruptions.

Diagnosis
- Unless considered in the differential diagnosis of skin disease on a regular basis, adverse drug reactions will be missed.

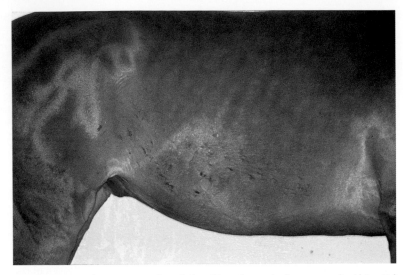

Figure 4.6 Papulocrustous rash with focal hair loss, which appeared within 48 h of administration of penicillin after a surgical procedure.

- The diagnosis can be based upon supportive medical history, ruling out other possible conditions and supportive histopathological changes.

Treatment
- If a drug eruption is suspected, all medication should be withdrawn.
- When some sort of therapy is considered essential, an alternative drug chemically unrelated to current or recently used substances should be chosen.
- Resolution of lesions usually occurs within 10–14 days but may take months.
- Corticosteroids may provide only minimal relief.
- Future exposure to the suspect drug and related compounds should be avoided; intentional re-exposure to confirm a diagnosis may result in more serious reactions and is contraindicated.

CONGENITAL AND HEREDITARY CAUSES

Aplasia cutis congenita (Epitheliogenesis imperfecta)

Clinical features
- Epitheliogenesis imperfecta (aplasia cutis congenita) has been reported on a number of occasions and particularly in Standardbred foals, but critical evaluation suggests that in the majority of these animals the actual diagnosis was epidermolysis bullosa.

- True aplasia cutis congenita is a very rare, likely inherited, condition characterised by full thickness skin defects, often of the distal limbs and face. Affected areas bleed easily and secondary infection is a common complication.

Diagnosis
- History and clinical signs.
- Nikolsky sign (separation of superficial epidermis on application of firm, sliding pressure to the skin) is absent.
- Biopsies from the edge of lesions reveal a complete absence of epidermis and epidermal appendages.
- The main differential apart from epidermolysis bullosa is obstetric trauma.

Treatment
- Small lesions may heal by scar formation or may be treated by surgical debridement and suturing or skin grafting.
- Affected sires and dams should be removed from breeding programmes.

Epidermolysis bullosa

Clinical features
- Epidermolysis bullosa (EB) encompasses a group of hereditary diseases characterised by blister formation at the dermo-epidermal junction following minor trauma.
- The disease in horses has been most commonly described in the Belgian draught breed and also in two French draught breeds, all sharing common ancestors. The condition is caused by an autosomal recessive genetic defect of a subunit of laminin 5, an anchoring filament in the lamina lucida of the basement membrane zone. The same genetic defect has been described in other breeds. In the American Standardbred the condition is due to a genetic defect in a different subunit of laminin 5. A genetic test is available; heterozygous carrier status of at least 30% has been reported in the Belgian draught breed and 5% in Standardbreds. Rarely, other congenital structural defects of the basement membrane zone have been reported.
- Signs:
  - Lesions are present at birth or occur shortly afterwards, affecting mucocutaneous junctions, oral mucosa, coronary bands, and skin over bony prominences.
  - Primary lesions are vesicles and bullae, but these easily rupture and the predominant presentation is well-demarcated ulcers; collapsed bullae may be seen on the oral mucosa.

- Coronary band lesions result in separation of the hoof capsules.
- Dystrophic teeth are common.

Diagnosis
- A positive Nikolsky sign can usually be elicited.
- The presence of characteristic lesions in a neonatal Belgian draught foal is clinically diagnostic.
- Histopathology:
  - Separation is evident at the dermo-epidermal junction, below the basal epithelium.
  - In junctional EB associated with laminin 5 defects, the separation leaves the PAS-positive staining basement membrane on the floor of the defect, attached to the dermis.

Treatment
- There is no treatment; the condition is fatal and euthanasia is indicated.
- Sire and dam should be removed from breeding programmes.
- Genetic testing of prospective stud animals is recommended to identify heterozygous carriers; testing available in both Europe (Center for Animal Genetics; www.centerforanimalgenetics.com/services/horse-genetic-testing/hereditary-disease-testing-for-horses) and North America (Veterinary Genetics Laboratory, University of California Davis; www.vgl.ucdavis.edu/services/horse).

Cutaneous asthenia (Hereditary equine regional dermal asthenia HERDA; Ehlers-Danlos syndrome)

Clinical features
- This disease has been reported in American Quarter horses and rarely in other breeds.
- The condition affects collagen synthesis and is apparent at birth or shortly thereafter, usually before 4 years of age. The genetic defect has been characterised in the Quarter horse breed; it is an autosomal recessive mutation that affects protein folding of collagen.
- Although lesions may appear localised or regional, the weakness of the skin is generalised; thus, the popular term 'hereditary equine regional dermal asthenia' (HERDA) is not biomechanically accurate.
- Signs:
  - Lesions may be solitary or multiple and commonly affect the dorsum and less commonly the neck, limbs, face.

- Areas of loose skin several inches in diameter are found, easily tented, and wrinkled and hyperextensible.
- The skin is fragile, tears easily, and heals poorly. In good light, the centre of lesions appears depressed. Pressure or traction applied at the edge of lesions may be painful.
- Occasionally, the presenting complaint is haematoma formation.
- Joint hypermobility does not appear to be a feature.

Diagnosis
- Characteristic lesions in a young Quarter horse are sufficiently diagnostic.
- Skin biopsies should be excisional rather than punch biopsies so that the full thickness of the dermis is included. Light microscopy may reveal greatly reduced or absence of deep dermal collagen layers, thinning of the dermis, fragmentation, and disorientation of collagen fibres.

Treatment
- There is no treatment.
- Trauma should be minimised.
- Lesions may heal with supportive therapy, but leave unsightly scars.
- Affected and related animals should not be used for breeding. Genetic testing is available (Veterinary Genetics Laboratory, University of California Davis; www.vgl.ucdavis.edu/services/horse; Center for Animal Genetics; www.centerforanimalgenetics.com/services/horse-genetic-testing/hereditary-disease-testing-for-horses; Laboklin UK; https://www.laboklin.co.uk/laboklin/showGeneticTest.jsp?testID=8139).

Warmblood fragile foal syndrome

Clinical features
- A similar condition affecting a different protein involved in collagen biosynthesis, analogous to human Ehlers-Danlos syndrome type IV, occurs in warmbloods, but has also been reported in other breeds. A low frequency of carrier status has been reported in Thoroughbreds.
- This lethal autosomal recessive disease affects the connective tissues of skin, mucosae, and joints; most affected foals are not carried to term and are spontaneously aborted or stillborn.

- Newborn foals show extensive skin separation, tearing, and ulceration resulting from minimal external trauma, without haemorrhage, ulcers on the gums and mucous membranes, and hypermobile joints (Figure 4.7); they may remain recumbent or make only weak attempts to stand.

Diagnosis

- Characteristic clinical signs in a neonatal foal may be diagnostic.
- Genetic testing is available for confirmation, and to detect carrier animals (Veterinary Genetics Laboratory, University of California Davis; Center for Animal Genetics; www.centerforanimalgenetics. com/services/horse-genetic-testing/hereditary-disease-testing-for-horses; Animal Genetics UK: https://www.animalgenetics.eu/Equine/Genetic_Disease/WFFS.asp).

Treatment

- Affected foals carried to term will not survive; euthanasia on humane grounds is indicated.
- Heterozygote carriers should not be used for breeding.

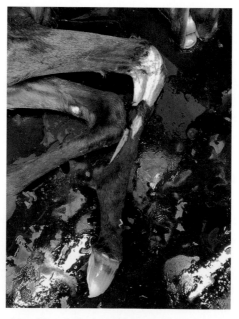

Figure 4.7 Warmblood fragile foal syndrome: extensive ulceration on the forelimbs of a neonatal foal homozygous for the PLOD1 gene. Source: Courtesy of Andrew McGladdery and Emily Floyd.

Hoof wall separation disease (HWSD)

Clinical features

- Recessive genetic defect of Connemara ponies; carrier frequency estimated at approximately 15%.
- Signs:
  - Fissures, cracks, and fractures in dorsal hoof wall originating at weight bearing surface.
  - Signs become apparent within first year of life.
  - Coronary band appears normal.
  - Proliferation of horn on sole of hooves.
  - Associated with signs of laminitis.
  - Variable severity; in severe cases, weight bearing on sole of foot with rotation of third phalanx results in severe lameness.

Diagnosis

- Genetic testing is available for confirmation, and to detect carrier animals (Veterinary Genetics Laboratory, University of California Davis; www.vgl.ucdavis.edu/services/horse; Center for Animal Genetics; www.centerforanimalgenetics.com/services/horse-genetic-testing/hereditary-disease-testing-for-horses).
- Differential diagnosis includes white line disease, laminitis, solar abscessation.

Treatment

- Frequent trimming of hooves, use of glue on shoes as use of nails results in splitting of horn.
- Euthanasia on humane grounds is indicated in severe cases.
- All registered Connemaras are required to be genetically tested and results recorded in passports.
- Heterozygote carriers should not be used for breeding.

ENVIRONMENTAL CAUSES

Burns

Clinical features

- Burns may result from thermal and chemical insults. Lesions may be classified according to the depth and severity of tissue damage.
- Signs:
  - First-degree burns present with erythema, superficial oedema, and marked pain, and resolve after superficial scaling.

- Second-degree burns show hair loss, superficial blistering, and epidermal necrosis with pain. Healing occurs in 7–10 days with no permanent damage.
- Third-degree burns have severe blistering with loss of the epidermis and superficial dermis and absence of pain except at the edge of lesions. Healing is slow and scarring ensues with an atrophic epidermis and loss of epidermal appendages.
- Fourth-degree burns involve loss of full-skin thickness and involve deeper tissues. Serious scarring and impairment of function follows prolonged healing.
- Assessment of the depth of lesions may be aided by insertion of a needle in the centre of lesions to gauge the presence of pain.
  - Superficial burns will retain an intact pain response.
  - Absence of a pain response indicates deeper tissue damage, with loss of the epidermis and superficial dermis including the cutaneous pain receptors.
- Considerable loss of plasma protein may accompany second-, third-, and fourth-degree burns involving large areas of the body; secondary infection is common.

Diagnosis
- History and clinical signs.

Treatment
- Early application of cold water for 20 minutes will limit further tissue damage.
- Intravenous fluid therapy may be required and broad-spectrum antibiotic cover may be indicated for second- and third-degree burns.
- Analgesia and sedation are indicated prior to wound cleansing, debridement, and dressing.
- Where possible, non-adherent semi-occlusive dressings should be applied. Skin grafting may be indicated.
- If burns are extensive or the depth of tissue damage is likely to result in functional impairment, or if there is ocular and lung involvement, then euthanasia may be indicated.

Tack and harness rubs and pressure sores

Clinical features
- The nature of lesions resulting from mechanical damage depends on the severity and duration of frictional forces applied:

- Sudden or sustained application of a considerable force such as results from a badly fitting harness or tack may result in erosions or ulceration of the skin, with exudation.
- Milder pressure or low-grade forces applied repeatedly induce hair loss, erythema, hyperkeratosis, and skin thickening or callus formation (Figure 4.8) In some cases, a dermal reaction occurs, sometimes without overlying hair loss, producing so-called 'corns' or 'sit-fasts'.
- Prolonged direct pressure, particularly over bony prominences, may result in ischaemic damage and even epidermal sloughing. Incorrectly applied limb bandages are often to blame.
- Scar tissue with an atrophic epithelium and absence of hair may ensue or the production of non-pigmented hair, if damage is less severe (Figure 4.9). These changes are typified by saddle sores.

Diagnosis
- History and clinical signs.

Treatment
- The cause of the damage must be identified and removed. In particular, the fit and padding of the saddle should be attended to in cases of dorsal lesions.
- Most minor lesions will resolve given sufficient time.
- Ischaemic changes and scar formation are permanent.
- Surgery for removal of corns or sit-fasts should be considered a last resort and may cause even greater problems.

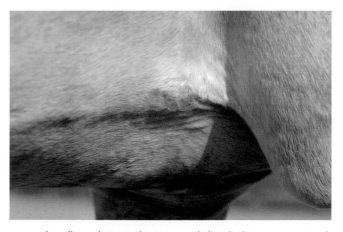

Figures 4.8   Girth gall: erythema, alopecia, and skin thickening associated with pressure from the girth or surcingle. Source: Courtesy of R.J. Payne.

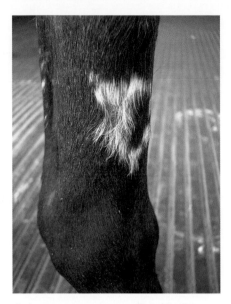

Figure 4.9   Area of alopecic scarring surrounded by non-pigmented hair (leucotrichia) as a sequel of inappropriate bandaging. Source: Courtesy of R.J. Payne.

Thrush

Clinical features
- A necrotic condition of the horn of the frog, affecting the sulci and may extend to involve the whole of the frog.
- Moist, wet environmental conditions predispose the horn of the frog to keratolytic anaerobic bacterial and fungal infection, most frequently involving *Fusobacterium necrophorum*.
- Signs:
    - More prevalent in hind feet than fore, but may occur in any one or more feet.
    - Distinctive foul odour when foot is examined.
    - Affected sulci have a thick, black, moist, malodorous discharge.
    - Probing may show the sulcus to be deeper than normal and may elicit haemorrhage.
    - Sloughing of necrotic horn of the frog (Figure 4.10).
    - Lameness absent in most cases unless advanced and involving deeper structures of the foot.

Diagnosis
- Clinical signs of characteristic black discharge and malodour.

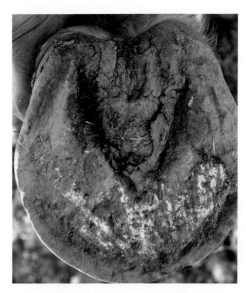

Figure 4.10 Thrush: loss of frog horn, ulceration, and fissuring with black necrotic material in the central and lateral sulci due to anaerobic infection. Source: Courtesy of Kieran O'Brien.

Treatment
- Improve stable management; ensure clean, dry underfoot environment.
- Regular foot hygiene.
- Initial debridement and daily application of antimicrobial solution until tissue returns to normality; antiseptic solutions containing chlorhexidine, iodine, and dilute bleach are effective. Systemic antibiosis is rarely necessary.
- Astringents may be useful.
- May require special shoeing.

NEOPLASTIC CAUSES

See Chapter 5.

MISCELLANEOUS DERMATOSES

Actinic dermatoses

Ultraviolet (UV) light can damage the skin acutely or chronically. To inflict damage, radiation must be absorbed by the skin, and this is facilitated by absence of, or a thin, haircoat and lack of pigment. Absorbed light results in molecular and biochemical changes including release of free radicals, with consequent damage to cellular structure and function. Acute damage can be phototoxic, which is dose-related and wavelength-related, or due to photosensitisation.

Phototoxicity
Sunburn

Clinical features
- Seen in cream or albino horses and animals with non-pigmented faces exposed to sunlight at peak intensity during the middle of summer days.
- Severity of damage is dose-related and wavelength-related; UVB light penetrates less deeply but is of higher energy than UVA light.
- Early changes consist of erythema due to dilatation of superficial vessels; damage allowing leakage of fluid results in swelling and blister formation, which progresses to erosion, ulceration, and crusting (Figure 4.11), followed by scaling, and alopecia (Figure 4.12).
- Prolonged exposure results in thickening and hyperkeratosis (Figure 4.13) and chronically may result in pre-malignant changes of actinic keratosis and ultimately neoplastic disease (see Chapter 5).

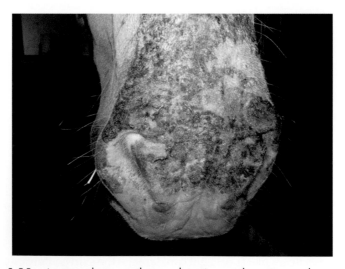

Figure 4.11   Acute sunburn: erythema, ulceration, and crusting on the muzzle of a horse kept at permanent pasture; note the abrupt demarcation between affected and unaffected, pigmented, skin. Source: Courtesy of A. Cox.

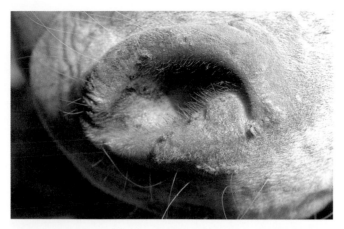

Figure 4.12 Sunburnt external naris showing erythema, scaling, and alopecia.

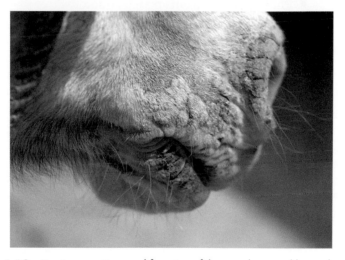

Figure 4.13 Erosion, crusting, and fissuring of the muzzle caused by sunburn.

Diagnosis

- History and clinical signs.
- Absence of liver pathology evident in blood biochemistry profiles.
- Histopathology reveals clusters of vacuolated keratinocytes (sunburn cells) in the superficial dermis, superficial vascular dilatation, spongiosis and oedema, depletion of Langerhans' cells and mast cells and a superficial neutrophilic to mixed dermal inflammation; in severe cases vesicles, bullae, and ulcers are seen with overlying crusts.

Treatment

- Appropriate supportive symptomatic therapy.
- Topical corticosteroid creams and non-steroidal anti-inflammatory (NSAID) drugs may be indicated.
- Prevent further exposure to sunlight until healed.
- Prevention by use of high factor (30–55 SPF) sunscreen and avoiding exposure to sunlight between 9 a.m. to 3 p.m. from spring to autumn.

Photosensitisation

Clinical features

- Photosensitisation requires the following:
  - Presence of a photodynamic agent within the skin.
  - Exposure to sufficient amount of UVA and UVB light.
  - Cutaneous absorption of this UV radiation.
- Photodynamic agents may be phototoxic or photoallergic.
- Phototoxic agents are capable of causing damage in nearly all animals.
- Photoallergy requires previous sensitisation and, whilst it is well recognised in humans, it is poorly understood in horses.
- Photodynamic agents may reach the skin by systemic or contact routes.
- Energy is absorbed by the photodynamic molecules and released into the tissues causing damage, primarily to the epidermis and superficial dermal blood vessels.
- Skin lesions are similar in all types of photosensitisation, although may differ in distribution:
  - Erythema, oedema, scaling, exudation and crusting, ulceration, necrosis, and sloughing.
  - Glabrous and poorly haired, non-pigmented skin affected; may extend to lightly pigmented and haired skin.

Contact photosensitisation

Clinical features

- Most cases have occurred in horses grazing lush pastures containing clover. Other plants including giant hogweed (*Heracleum mantegazzianum*) can also cause contact photosensitisation.
- The mechanisms are poorly understood, but may involve either phototoxic or photoallergic responses to absorbed photodynamic molecules. Involvement of multiple animals on a pasture indicates phototoxicity rather than a hypersensitivity immunological mechanism.
- Signs:
  - Only areas of contact are involved, and lesions are restricted to non-pigmented areas of the muzzle and lips and the distal extremities.

Primary systemic photosensitisation

Clinical features

- Ingestion of plants or drugs containing photodynamic compounds which are absorbed and reach the skin via the circulation. Subsequent exposure to sufficient UV radiation results in cutaneous lesions in light-skinned regions of the body.
- Many plants may cause systemic photosensitisation including St John's wort, perennial ryegrass, Alsike clover, buckwheat, and brassicas.
- The photodynamic chemical involved has not been identified in all cases and it is not understood why the incidence of photosensitisation may vary on the same pasture from year to year.
- Drugs and chemicals that are photosensitising include phenothiazines, thiazides, methylene blue, sulphonamides, tetracyclines, and coal tar derivatives.
- Signs:
  - Lesions are most severe on thinly haired, non-pigmented areas such as muzzle, lips, eyelids, but may affect non-pigmented haired

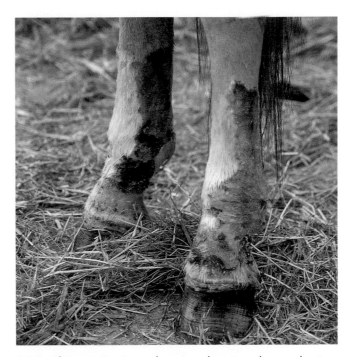

Figure 4.14 Photosensitisation: alopecia, ulceration, haemorrhagic exudation, necrosis, and sloughing of the non-pigmented distal limbs of a pony out at grass. Several animals in the group were affected, with no evidence of hepatic pathology, indicating primary photosensitisation. Source: Courtesy of S.C. Shaw.

skin anywhere on the body and occasionally extend to lightly pigmented skin (Figure 4.14).
- Multiple animals grazed on the same pasture are usually affected. Where photoallergic mechanisms are involved, only a single individual may be affected.

Secondary (hepatogenous) photosensitisation

Clinical features

- Animals with liver disease have impaired ability to excrete the photodynamic agent phylloerythrin, which is produced by bacterial fermentation of chlorophyll. Phylloerythrin may accumulate in the tissues resulting in photosensitisation.
- Hepatotoxins that may cause secondary photosensitisation include alkaloids and saponins found in various plants, but the most commonly implicated is ragwort (*Senecio jacobaea*). This is a notifiable weed in some countries, but nevertheless is widespread on roadside verges and over-grazed pastures. Horses avoid ingesting the plant when it is growing in pasture, but may consume significant quantities in hay gathered from fields where the plant is present.
- Mycotoxins in water containing blue-green algae are hepatotoxic.
- Other liver diseases may also result in impaired biliary excretion of phylloerythrin and signs of photosensitisation.
- Signs are identical to primary photosensitisation but tend to affect individuals or small numbers of animals rather than all animals grazing in a field.

Diagnosis of photosensitisation

- Lesions are usually limited to the non-pigmented skin of grazing animals.
- Number of animals affected and lesion distribution should give a clue to the type of photosensitivity involved.
- Liver function tests should be run on all cases, even when multiple animals are involved, since all animals may have been exposed to an agent causing hepatic damage.
- Skin biopsy not usually necessary; changes depend on stage of disease, with epidermal and dermal oedema, vacuolated and apoptotic keratinocytes, and superficial dermal vascular changes seen in early lesions and diffuse necrotising or fibrosing dermatitis in older lesions.

Treatment

- Prevent exposure to sunlight by stabling.
- Further exposure to the photodynamic agent should be prevented.

- Corticosteroids used early in the course of the disease will reduce inflammation.
- NSAIDs may be indicated.
- Symptomatic topical therapy to cool and soothe.
- Systemic antibiotics may be required.
- Surgical debridement of necrotic and sloughing tissue may be required.
- Appropriate supportive therapy for liver disease.
- Prognosis for primary photosensitisation is usually favourable but guarded to poor in hepatogenous cases.

Hepatocutaneous syndrome (superficial necrolytic dermatitis)

Clinical features
- Metabolic disturbances associated with severe liver pathology can result in skin lesions, particularly affecting mucocutaneous and skin-horn junctions.
- Signs include ulceration of lips, muzzle, oral mucosa, coronary bands, chestnuts and ergots; patchy hair loss is also seen at sites affected by serum exudation.

Diagnosis
- Liver enzymes and bile acids markedly elevated.
- Biopsies show characteristic changes of epidermal hyperplasia with spongiosis and marked parakeratosis, crusting, and areas of ulceration, accompanied by a hyperplastic, mixed, perivascular dermatitis; secondary bacterial infection may be present.

Treatment
- Supportive therapy may secure temporary amelioration of clinical signs, but the prognosis is poor to grave since the underlying liver pathology is not usually amenable to treatment.

REFERENCES AND FURTHER READING

Barlaam, A., Traversa, D., Papini, R. et al. (2020) Habronematidosis in equids: Current status, advances, future challenges. *Frontiers in Veterinary Science*, 7: 358.

Equine Genetic Disease Testing: Animal Genetics UK. https://www.animalgenetics.eu/Equine/Genetic_Disease/Disease_Index.asp

Scott, D. and Miller, W. (2011). *Equine Dermatology (2nd edition)*. Maryland Heights, MO: W.B. Saunders Company.

University of California Davis Veterinary Genetics Laboratory Index of Equine DNA tests. https://vgl.ucdavis.edu/tests?field_species_target_id=266

Papules, Nodules, and Masses 5

Nodular diseases form a sizeable component of equine dermatology. Papules are circumscribed, elevated lesions up to 1 cm in diameter; nodules are circumscribed, elevated, solid lesions up to 2 cm in diameter; larger lesions may be termed masses. Important factors to consider are age of onset, speed of onset, breed, seasonality, and history of systemic disease or recent treatment (Figure 5.1).

Clinical examination is necessary to assess the presence of systemic disease, number of lesions, location on the body surface, signs of injury or trauma, presence of discharge, and pain or pruritus. Needle aspirates, impression smears, and microbial culture are often indicated but, in most cases, histopathology is necessary for definitive diagnosis.

PHYSICAL CONDITIONS

Haematoma

Clinical features
- Traumatic event preceding development of subcutaneous swelling.
- May see discoloration of skin.
- Swelling may be variably firm to hard (Figure 5.2).

Diagnosis
- History of trauma, physical appearance, skin may pit on pressure.
- Ultrasound examination of swelling.

Practical Equine Dermatology, Second Edition. Janet D. Littlewood, David H. Lloyd and J. Mark Craig.
© 2022 John Wiley & Sons Ltd. Published 2022 by John Wiley & Sons Ltd.

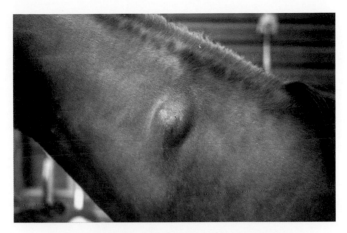

Figure 5.1 Injection abscess. Source: Courtesy of Andrew Browning.

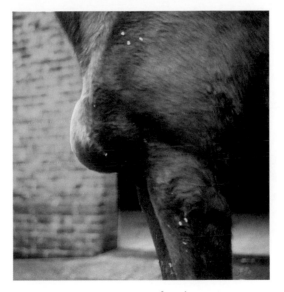

Figure 5.2 Haematoma. Source: Courtesy of Andrew Browning.

- Needle aspiration to confirm presence of blood, or serum in an organising haematoma.
- Consider coagulopathy (e.g. haemophilia A) in cases of large haematoma or multiple haematomata with only minimal trauma; check platelet count, activated clotting time, one-stage prothrombin time, activated partial thromboplastin time.
- Differentials: abscess, neoplasia, cyst, urticaria.

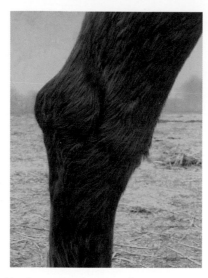

Figure 5.3   Capped hock. Source: Courtesy of Kieran O'Brien.

Treatment
- Hot and cold compresses.
- Rest.

Bursitis

Clinical features
- Enlargement and inflammation of a bursa overlying a tendon or joint.
- Often occurs over the point of the elbow or hock ('capped hock') (Figure 5.3).
- Swelling may be variably soft to firm.

Diagnosis
- Clinical appearance.
- Ultrasonography.
- Needle aspiration, after rigorous aseptic preparation of the site.
- Differentials: abscess, bruising, haematoma, calcinosis circumscripta, enlarged joint capsule, neoplasia.

Treatment
- Pressure bandages.
- Drainage.

- Glucocorticoids in non-infected cases.
- Surgical drainage or removal.

Hernia/rupture

Clinical features
- Herniation occurs at sites of natural anatomical 'openings'; ruptures are splits or tears in muscle sheaths or between muscle planes allowing protrusion of muscle or abdominal contents.
- Common sites are scrotal, inguinal, or umbilical (Figure 5.4), or at sites where muscle injury causes loss of restraint by normal muscle sheath. May occur as a complication of castration or laparotomy.
- Signs:
    - Swelling in areas known to be associated with herniation or at sites of previous injury or surgical incision.

Diagnosis
- History and clinical appearance.
- Ultrasonography.
- Needle aspiration, with care.
- Surgical exploration.
- Differentials: abscess, haematoma, scirrhous cord, neoplasia.

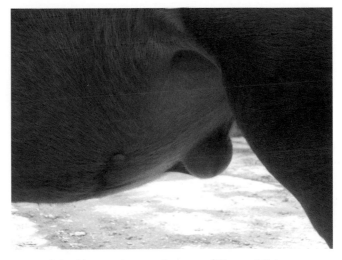

Figure 5.4 Umbilical hernia. Source: Courtesy of Kieran O'Brien.

Treatment
• Surgical reduction and repair.

CYSTS

Cysts are cavities lined with epithelium, containing fluid or solid material. They present as smooth, well-circumscribed, fluctuant to solid nodules or masses.

Follicular cyst

Clinical features
• Uncommon, classified according to part of follicle from which cyst arises:
  – Infundibular.
  – Isthmus (trichilemmal).
  – Matrical (pilar).
• May be congenital or acquired due to damage to the follicle.
• Usually solitary lesions, soft to firm, well-circumscribed, found mostly on head or distal limbs.
• May progressively enlarge due to continuing exfoliation of keratinised material.
• Overlying skin is usually normal.

Diagnosis
• Clinical findings.
• Ultrasonography.
• Fine needle aspirate:
  – Many squames, occasional cholesterol crystals in oily background material; no evidence of inflammation or infection.
• Contents are yellow-grey mucoid to greasy material.
• Histologically most arise from the follicular infundibulum, with a differentiated epithelial lining and containing layers of keratin.
• Differentials: abscess, foreign body, fistula, other cysts, neoplasia.

Treatment
• Surgical excision.
• Monitor without treatment.
• Prognosis:
  – Unlikely to resolve without therapy.

Atheroma (epidermoid cyst, epithelial inclusion cyst)

Clinical features
- Subcutaneous nodule found unilaterally (rarely bilaterally) in or over the false nostril; congenital, but may not become apparent until the horse is 3–6 months old.
- Does not usually cause respiratory noise or obstruction.
- Likely to be a form of infundibular follicular cyst.
- May continue to enlarge slowly over time.

Diagnosis
- As for other follicular cysts (see above).

Treatment
- As for other follicular cysts (see above).

Dermoid cysts

Clinical features
- Uncommon, resulting from embryonic displacement of ectoderm into the subcutis.
- Seen at birth or during first year of life; may be hereditary.
- Cysts contain hair, keratin, and secretions from sebaceous and sweat glands.
- Signs:
  - Firm, well-circumscribed, single or multiple non-painful nodules.
  - Found on dorsal midline, with normal overlying skin.

Diagnosis
- Clinical findings.
- Ultrasonography.
- Fine needle aspirates reveal squames in oily material.
- Histology:
  - Differentiated epithelial lining with well-developed small hair follicles and sebaceous glands, occasional sweat glands.
  - Lumen contains keratin and hair shafts.

Treatment
- Leave and monitor.
- Surgical excision.
- Prognosis:
  - Unlikely to resolve without therapy.

Heterotopic polyodontia (conchal/periauricular) cyst

Clinical features
- Rare developmental defect due to aberrant tooth germ arising from the first branchial arch.
- Often incorrectly termed 'dentigerous cyst'.
- Congenital, but may not be recognised until adulthood.
- Signs:
  - Fluctuant, non-painful swelling at the base of the ear (Figure 5.5).
  - Solitary, occasionally bilateral.
  - May discharge a mucoid, milky secretion.

Diagnosis
- History and clinical signs.
- Ultrasonography.
- Fine needle aspirate.
- Radiography may reveal tooth-like structures.
- Histopathological findings:
  - Fistula with epidermal lining including hair follicles and adnexa.
  - Ectopic teeth or tooth-like structures.
- Differentials: abscess, foreign body, other cysts, neoplasia.

Treatment
- Leave and monitor.
- Surgical excision.

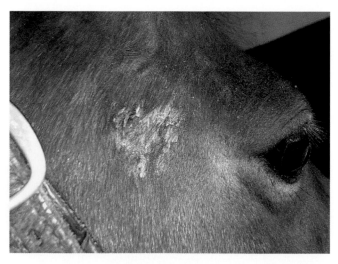

Figure 5.5 Heterotopic polyodontia (periauricular cyst) with seepage of mucoid material from fistula.

- Prognosis:
  - Unlikely to resolve without therapy.

VIRAL CONDITIONS

Viral papillomatosis (warts)

Clinical features
- Common condition of horses under 3 years of age, no age or breed predisposition.
- Caused by equine papillomavirus (*Equus caballus* papillomavirus, EcPV) transmitted by direct or indirect contact; seven EcPV types have been characterised, type 1 being the principal agent in classical papillomatosis.
- Infection requires damaged skin, e.g. trauma, insect or ectoparasite bite, ultraviolet light damage.
- Incubation period 19–67 days.
- Signs:
  - Usually multiple, raised, verrucous proliferations of epidermis.
  - Variable lesion size, 1 mm to 2 cm, greyish-white to pink in colour, with hyperkeratotic surface.
  - Lesions are non-pruritic and non-painful.
  - Most commonly seen around the eyes (Figure 5.6), muzzle (Figure 5.7), lips, distal limbs, external genitalia.

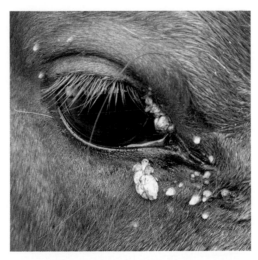

Figure 5.6 Viral papillomata affecting the periocular region of a Thoroughbred yearling. Source: Courtesy of Oliver Pynn.

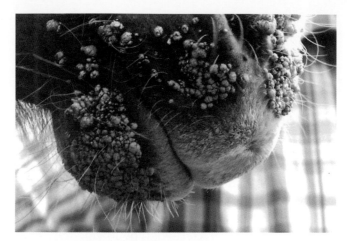

Figure 5.7 Papillomata affecting the muzzle in a 2-year-old. Source: Courtesy of S. Bjornson.

Diagnosis
- Age of onset, site, and clinical appearance of lesions.
- Biopsy for confirmation not usually necessary:
  - Features include epidermal hyperplasia, acanthosis, papillomatosis, parakeratotic hyperkeratosis, koilocytes (perinuclear halos), clumping of keratohyalin granules, and intranuclear inclusion bodies.
  - Papillomavirus antigen can be demonstrated by immunohistochemistry.
- Differentials: sarcoid, horse pox, molluscum contagiosum, epidermal hamartoma/nevus.

Treatment
- Spontaneous resolution usually occurs within 2–3 months, mediated by cellular immunity, which is usually lifelong.
- Persistent lesions may be removed surgically or with cryotherapy.
- Topical agents licensed for treatment of warts in humans may be useful, used off-label:
  - Podophyllotoxin 0.15% cream (Warticon, Phoenix Labs) applied to lesions twice daily for 3 consecutive days of the week prevents cellular division and causes subsequent death of wart tissue.
  - Imiquimod 5% cream (Aldara, Meda Pharmaceuticals; Bascellex, Ranbaxy UK) applied to lesions on 3 days of the week; wash off after 6–10 hours; up-regulates local production of interferon.

- Prognosis is usually good, but where lesions persist for more than 12 months, immune compromise should be suspected.
- Prevention:
  - Isolate infected horses.
  - Prevent exposure of naive horses to infected pastures and premises.
  - Disinfect feeding, grooming, and tack equipment.
- Autogenous vaccines may elicit a humoral antibody response, and there is recent published evidence of therapeutic benefit.

Aural plaques

Clinical features
- Common disease of adult horses, over 1 year of age; four types of EcPV have been detected in lesions, −3, −4, −5, and −6.
- No sex or breed predisposition.
- Transmission thought to be associated with black flies, *Simulium* spp.; condition is not seen in regions such as New Zealand where these flies are absent.
- Signs:
  - Lesions consist of greyish-white, alopecic papules which coalesce to form hyperkeratotic plaques (Figure 5.8) affecting the concave surface of the pinna, bilaterally or unilaterally.
  - Usually no associated discomfort, although interference with lesions may result in head-shy behaviour.

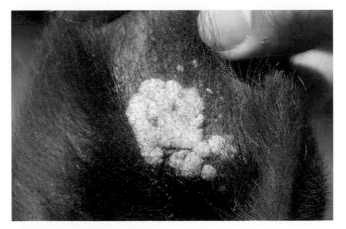

Figure 5.8 Aural plaques. Depigmented hyperkeratotic plaques on the concave surface of the pinna.

Diagnosis
- Gross appearance and location of lesions is characteristic.
- Biopsy for histopathology and immunohistochemistry not usually necessary.

Treatment
- Leave alone as of cosmetic concern only.
- Application of imiquimod 5% cream (off-label use; Aldara, Meda Pharmaceuticals) shown to be effective in resolution of high proportion of lesions, but requires months of treatment and may cause irritation, crusting, and inflammation.
- Prognosis:
  - Lesions tend to persist indefinitely.
  - Rarely may progress to squamous cell carcinoma.

Genital papilloma

Clinical features
- Proliferative lesions caused by EcPV-2 can affect the external genitalia of both male and female horses.
- Transmission may be venereal, but lesions can also affect geldings, and mares and stallions that have never bred, so transmission by fomites and insects is proposed.
- Population studies suggest a prevalence of seroconversion in approximately one-third of animals, but a lower prevalence of viral DNA detection (less than 20%).
- Lesions may progress to pre-cancerous plaques and squamous cell carcinoma (SCC).
- Signs:
  - Small, papillomatous or plaque-like lesions, progressing to larger cauliflower-like or pedunculated lesions.
  - Can affect any part of genital epithelium but most commonly found on glans and free part of the penis of males (Figure 5.9) and vulva of mares.
  - Seen in older horses; no strong evidence of breed predisposition.
  - Male horses may show preputial oedema, dysuria, haematuria, urinary incontinence, and weight loss associated with malignant transformation.

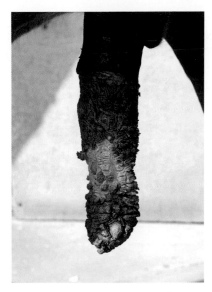

Figure 5.9   Genital papillomata. Hyperkeratotic proliferative papules diffusely affecting the shaft and glans of the penis.

Diagnosis
- Biopsy for histological examination:
  - Well-differentiated epithelial papillomata with progressive squamous differentiation and keratinisation.
  - Areas of disordered epithelial differentiation and keratinisation, epidermal dysplasia, anisokaryosis (variable nuclear size), and mitoses with an intact basement membrane are consistent with carcinoma in situ.
  - Penetration of epithelial cells into the submucosa is indicative of invasive SCC.
- Differentials include sarcoids, habronemiasis, granulomata, non-specific balanoposthitis.

Treatment
- Topical treatment of penile lesions can be considered, but is difficult and likely to lead to unacceptable inflammation and discomfort.
- See below for treatment of SCC.
- Prognosis is guarded as papillomatous lesions may progress to malignant transformation and although penile SCC has low metastatic potential, involvement of drainage lymph nodes and occasionally distant metastasis may occur.

- Prevention:
  - No proven guidelines as the method of transmission is not certain.
  - Careful hygiene precautions when cleaning external genitalia.
  - Prophylactic vaccine containing virus-like particles (VLP) may become available.

Molluscum contagiosum

Clinical features

- Caused by a molluscipox virus with close homology to the virus causing the disease in humans; may represent an anthropozoonosis with transmission from human to animal. Disease in humans is associated with immunocompromise and this may be involved in equine cases.
- Signs:
  - Papular lesions begin in one body region, becoming widespread, affecting neck, shoulders, chest, limbs, but occasionally remaining more localised.
  - Tufted lesions in haired skin, which become alopecic with powdery crusts and scale (Figure 5.10).
  - Some papules develop a central pore with a whitish to brown projection.

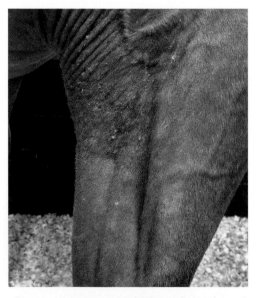

Figure 5.10 Molluscum contagiosum. Multiple small papules with central white core or plug in the axillary region of a horse with concurrent pituitary pars intermedia dysfunction (PPID). Source: Courtesy of Celia Marr.

- Coalescence of lesions may result in plaques or proliferative nodules.
- Lesions sometimes ulcerate and bleed when traumatised.
- In non-haired areas lesions are waxy, umbilicated papules.
- Hyper- or hypopigmentation may occur as lesions heal (see Chapter 7).

Diagnosis
- Biopsy reveals well-demarcated epidermal hyperplasia and papillomatosis, swelling of keratinocytes with eosinophilic intracytoplasmic inclusion (molluscum) bodies, which become larger and basophilic as cells progress towards the skin surface, compressing the cell nucleus. Molluscum bodies are shed through the central pore.

Treatment
- No effective treatment is reported, and lesions may persist or wax and wane for long periods. Although full spontaneous resolution has not been described, one of the authors has seen a case in a horse with pituitary pars intermedia dysplasia (PPID) which showed marked improvement in lesions with treatment for the PPID.

BACTERIAL INFECTIONS

Folliculitis, furunculosis

See Chapter 3.

Cellulitis

Clinical features
- Poorly defined, severe, deep, suppurative infection involving the dermis and subcutaneous tissues.
- Rare, no age or sex predilection.
- Majority of reported cases are in thoroughbreds and racehorses.
- Cause:
  - Coagulase positive staphylococci in the great majority of cases.
  - *Streptococcus* spp., *Escherichia coli*, *Enterobacter* spp. and other organisms less commonly isolated.
  - Often no history of trauma or injury preceding onset of the condition.
- Signs:
  - Severe and painful swelling of one (often hind) limb with marked lameness.

- Pyrexia, distress, and tachycardia.
- Complications include necrosis, sloughing, laminitis of affected or contralateral limb, osteomyelitis, and bacteraemia.

Diagnosis

- Clinical presentation of acute onset of lameness, swelling, and pain.
- Ultrasound examination to support the clinical diagnosis and demonstrate the presence and location of fluid pockets for aspiration and drainage.
- Culture of aspirated exudate.
- Blood samples reveal leucocytosis, neutrophilia, hyperfibrinogenaemia, and elevated C-reactive protein.

Treatment

- Early initiation of aggressive systemic antibiosis, usually a combination of a beta-lactam drug and an aminoglycoside. Third-level antibiotics should be reserved for use where lower-level drugs are not appropriate, based on culture and sensitivity data. (See BEVA resources for veterinarians: Protect ME antimicrobial policy guidance, www.beva.org. uk//Portals/0/Documents/ResourcesForVets/1beva-antimicrobial-policy-template-distributed.pdf). The doses recommended below are as advised in the literature and in the guidance document, rather than those stated in the data sheets:
  - Procaine penicillin (Depocillin 300 mg/ml Solution, MSD Animal Health) 20,000–25,000 iu/kg (12–15 mg/kg) intramuscularly every 12 hours.
  - Gentamicin (Genta-Equine 100 mg/ml solution for injection, Dechra) 6.6 mg/kg intravenously every 24 hours.
  - Ceftiofur (Excenel, Zoetis) 2 mg/kg intramuscularly every 12 hours.
  - Enrofloxacin (Baytril Solution for Injection, Elanco UK AH) off-label use, 5 mg/kg intravenously every 24 hours.
- Antibiosis should continue until infection has completely resolved.
- Concurrent use of non-steroidal anti-inflammatory drugs.
- Support bandages on the affected and contralateral limb.
- Prognosis is guarded:
  - Up to 25% of horses require euthanasia on humane grounds.
  - Return to soundness and intended use reported in around 75% of discharged animals.
  - Recurrence may occur in around 25% of cases.

Abscesses

Clinical features
- Localised, fluctuant to firm lesions consisting of dead inflammatory cells, liquefied tissue, and debris.
- Caused by bacterial contamination of skin wounds and injection sites.
- Usually caused by *Corynebacterium pseudotuberculosis*.
- Less frequently *Clostridia* spp., various anaerobes, coagulase positive staphylococci, streptococci, *Trueperella* (formerly *Arcanobacterium*) *pyogenes*, *Actinomyces* spp., *Nocardia* spp., *Actinobacillus* spp., and *Rhodococcus equi*.
- Occasionally abscesses may be sterile.
- Signs:
  - Circumscribed subcutaneous accumulation of pus (Figure 5.1).

Diagnosis
- Clinical signs.
- Ultrasonography.
- Aspiration of purulent exudate, examination of stained smears, bacterial culture.
- Differentials include cysts, haematomata, mycetomata, neoplasia.

Treatment
- Hot compresses and, or, poultices to bring lesions to a head.
- Surgical drainage and debridement.
- Flushing and packing with antimicrobial agents.
- Systemic antibiotics based on sensitivity testing, not before the abscess matures.
- If clostridial species are involved, use aggressive drainage and high-dose antimicrobial therapy.
  - Sodium penicillin 20,000–25,000 iu/kg (12–15 mg/kg) intravenously every 6–8 hours (off-label use of human product Benzylpenicillin sodium, Genus Pharmaceuticals).
  - Metronidazole 15 mg/kg intravenously every 12 hours (off-label use of human product, Baxter Healthcare).
- Prognosis usually good.
  - In sites of poor drainage or involvement of clostridial species, prognosis is poor.
- Prevention by careful attention to wound hygiene and aseptic injection technique.

Strangles

Clinical features
- Acute, contagious, upper respiratory tract infection caused by *Streptococcus equi* subsp. *equi* with abscess formation in mandibular or retropharyngeal lymph nodes.
- Signs:
  - Pyrexia.
  - Mucopurulent nasal discharge with mandibular or retropharyngeal lymphadenopathy (Figure 5.11).
  - Ulceration of enlarged lymph nodes with purulent discharge.
  - Hypersensitivity mechanisms lead to vasculitis in some cases (see purpura haemorrhagica in Chapter 4).

Diagnosis
- Clinical signs; history of contact with infected animals.
- Cytological examination of exudate.
- Bacterial culture, PCR testing:
  - Sensitivity testing often not necessary because of the predictable antibiotic sensitivity of streptococci.
- Elevation of antibodies against the species-specific M protein (SeM) by ELISA is indicative of recent infection, but also seen after recent vaccination and in purpura haemorrhagica.

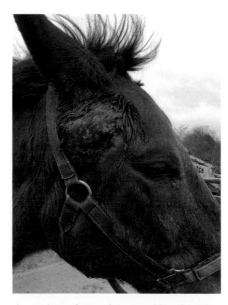

Figure 5.11 Strangles. Enlarged retropharyngeal lymph node on the point of rupture. Source: Courtesy of Kieran O'Brien.

Treatment
- Over 90% of streptococcal isolates are sensitive to penicillin, amoxicillin, cephalosporins, and trimethoprim-potentiated sulphonamides:
  - Procaine penicillin (Depocillin 300 mg/ml Solution, MSD Animal Health) 20,000–25,000 iu/kg (12–15 mg/kg) intramuscularly every 12 hours.
  - Trimethoprim-potentiated sulfadiazine (Trimediazine Powder/Oral Paste, Vetoquinol; Norodine Equine Oral Paste, Norbrook Laboratories) 30 mg/kg by mouth twice daily, every 12 hours.
- Hot compresses to encourage rupture of abscesses; surgical drainage.
- Isolation of infected horses.
- Quarantine new horses introduced to premises.
- For animals identified as being at risk, vaccination with a modified live strain of bacteria (Equilis Strep E, MSD Animal Health) confers protection on average in 75% of animals, but duration of immunity is only 3 months. Vaccine is administered by submucosal injection into the upper lip; no reversion to virulence has been seen and no transmission of the vaccinal strain to other horses.

Bacterial pseudomycetoma

Clinical features
- Uncommon granulomatous skin condition associated with chronic bacterial infection, often following wound contamination.
- Bacteria are present in tissues as granules (grains).
- Cause:
  - Actinomycotic mycetoma: *Nocardia*, and *Actinomyces* spp.
  - Other bacteria, e.g. *Actinobacillus*, staphylococci (botryomycosis), *Pseudomonas* spp.
- Signs:
  - Nodules, solitary or multiple, (Figure 5.12) often with ulceration and draining tracts.
  - Tissue granules usually visible in exudate.

Diagnosis
- Clinical signs.
- Microscopical examination of stained smears of needle aspirates, histopathological examination of biopsies, bacterial culture of aspirated exudate, and biopsy material.
- Differentials include fungal granulomata, habronemiasis, exuberant granulation tissue, neoplasia.

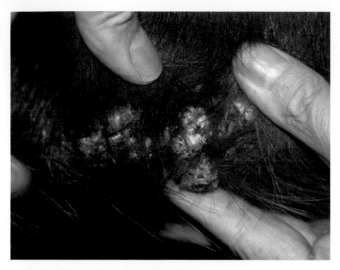

Figure 5.12 Nodular lesions of botryomycosis (*Staphylococcus aureus*), 1–2 cm diameter, with alopecia and crusting, along the mandible of a horse.

Treatment

- Prolonged systemic antibiotics based on culture and sensitivity:
  - Trimethoprim-potentiated sulfadiazine (Trimediazine Powder/ Oral Paste, Vetoquinol; Norodine Equine Oral Paste, Norbrook Laboratories) 30 mg/kg by mouth twice daily, every 12 hours.
  - Alternative oral drug is off-label use of doxycycline solution (Karidox 100 mg/ml solution for chicken and pigs, Nimrod Veterinary Products) 10 mg/kg by mouth every 12 hours.
  - Procaine penicillin (Depocillin 300 mg/ml Solution, MSD Animal Health) 20,000–25,000 iu/kg (12–15 mg/kg) intramuscularly every 12 hours, or with dihydrostreptomycin 20 mg/kg intramuscularly every 24 hours (Pen & Strep Suspension for Injection, Norbrook Laboratories; dose of 1 ml per 12.5 kg bodyweight).
  - Ceftiofur (Excenel, Zoetis) 2 mg/kg intramuscularly every 12 hours.
  - When no first- or second-generation drugs are suitable, enrofloxacin 100 mg/ml solution for poultry can be given (Baytril 10% Oral Solution, Elanco; Lanflox 100 mg/ml Solution, Nimrod; Enroxil 100 mg/ml Solution, Dechra) at a dose of 7.5 mg/kg once daily by mouth.
- Surgical excision or debulking may shorten time to resolution; antibiosis should continue until 2–4 weeks beyond clinical cure.

Ulcerative lymphangitis (epizootic lymphangitis)

Clinical features
- Bacterial infection of cutaneous lymphatics, now rare.
- Contamination of skin wounds, by direct contact or insect vectors.
- Cause:
  - *Corynebacterium pseudotuberculosis* is most commonly isolated.
  - Other organisms include staphylococci, streptococci, *Trueperella* (formerly *Arcanobacterium*) *pyogenes*, *Rhodococcus equi*, *Pasteurella haemolytica*, *Pseudomonas aeruginosa*, *Fusobacterium necrophorum*, and *Actinobacillus equuli*.
  - Mixed infections may occur.
- Signs:
  - Painful, hard to fluctuant, discharging nodules on distal hind limbs, may be unilateral or bilateral.
  - Draining tracts with creamy, greenish-white purulent exudate.
  - Regional lymphatics enlarged, hardened, and corded.
  - Lameness, pyrexia, lethargy, and anorexia often present.
  - Sometimes fatal.

Diagnosis
- Clinical signs.
- Stained smears, skin biopsies for culture, histopathology, and special stains:
  - Histological features are diffuse or nodular, suppurative to pyo-granulomatous dermatitis.
- Differentials: sporotrichosis, actinomycosis, nocardiosis, mycobacterial infections; also, glanders and histoplasmosis farciminosi in countries where these diseases occur.

Treatment
- Early and aggressive antimicrobial therapy, a beta-lactam drug alone or in conjunction with oral rifampicin until lameness and swelling improve:
  - Procaine penicillin (Depocillin 300 mg/ml Solution, MSD Animal Health) 20,000–25,000 iu/kg (12–15 mg/kg) intramuscularly every 12 hours, or with dihydrostreptomycin 20 mg/kg intramuscularly every 24 hours (Pen & Strep Suspension for Injection, Norbrook Laboratories; dose of 1 ml per 12.5 kg bodyweight).
  - Ceftiofur (Excenel, Zoetis) 2 mg/kg intramuscularly every 12 hours.
  - Rifampicin 5 mg/kg by mouth every 12 hours (off-label use of human drug; Rifadin, Sanofi; Rimactane, Sandoz).

- Continue treatment with oral trimethoprim-potentiated sulphona-mides until 2 weeks beyond clinical cure (often 1–2 months):
  - Trimethoprim-potentiated sulfadiazine (Trimediazine Powder/Oral Paste, Vetoquinol; Norodine Equine Oral Paste, Norbrook Laboratories) 30 mg/kg by mouth twice daily, every 12 hours.
- Hydrotherapy, lead exercise, leg wraps, and non-steroidal anti-inflammatory drugs.
- Good hygiene and management, early wound treatment, effective insect control.

Mycobacterial infections

Clinical features
- Skin lesions due to mycobacterial organisms are very rare.
- Cause:
  - Cutaneous tuberculosis caused by *Mycobacterium bovis* now extremely rare.
  - *M. avium* complex is the most common cause of mycobacterial skin lesions.
  - Opportunistic infections with atypical mycobacteria such as *M. smegmatis*.
- Signs:
  - Nodules, plaques, ulcers, draining tracts, abscess formation; may be painful.
  - Systemic signs may be present depending on other organ involvement:
    - weight loss, weakness, lethargy, stiffness, pyrexia, lymphade-nopathy, chronic cough, diarrhoea.

Diagnosis
- History of contact with infected animal, clinical signs.
- Skin biopsies for histopathological examination and special stains:
  - Granulomatous to pyogranulomatous dermatitis and panniculitis with variable numbers of acid-fast intracellular bacilli are seen.
- Submit tissue for mycobacterial culture and PCR to specialist laboratory.
- Tuberculin tests not useful as 70% of normal horses show positive intradermal reactions to purified mammalian and avian tuberculin.

Treatment
- Largely impractical due to expense of long-term drug administration.
- Euthanasia is the usual outcome.
- Occasionally. localised lesions may be excised; recovery from an abscess infected with the atypical mycobacterial species *M. smegmatis* has been reported.

Glanders (farcy)

Clinical features
- Notifiable, contagious, infectious, zoonotic fatal disease, seen in Asia, Africa, South America, and Eastern Europe.
- Caused by intracellular gram-negative bacillus *Burkholderia mallei*.
- Signs:
  - Acute and chronic forms of disease occur.
  - Acute disease – pyrexia, cough, nasal discharge, nodules, and ulcers affecting nasal mucosa and skin, painful lymphadenopathy, epistaxis, septicaemia, and death in days.
  - Chronic form more common in affected horses – insidious onset of malaise, weight loss, intermittent pyrexia, cough, nodular skin lesions, and in chains along lymphatics, lymphadenopathy. Nodules may ulcerate; nasal discharge and ulceration may develop. Affected horses may partially recover, becoming shedding carriers of disease, or may die.

Diagnosis
- Clinical signs of cutaneo-lymphatic disease with concurrent respiratory signs.
- Identification of organism in smears.
- Positive intradermal mallein test.
- Culture, serology, PCR.
- Differentials of other nodular diseases are rarely associated with respiratory disease.

Treatment
- Notify appropriate authorities.
- Euthanasia and safe disposal of carcase.

FUNGAL INFECTIONS

Dermatophytic pseudomycetoma

Clinical features
- Rare manifestation of *Trichophyton equinum* dermatophyte infection.
- Signs:
  - Dermal to subcutaneous nodules, single or multiple, may be ulcerated and discharge.
  - Lesions usually on dorsal thoracic trunk.

Diagnosis
- Smears of exudate may reveal fungal elements.
- Biopsy for histopathological examination, special stains, tissue culture:
  - Nodular to diffuse, granulomatous to pyogranulomatous panniculitis and dermatitis with folliculitis and furunculosis; fungal elements present as septate hyphae and arthroconidia in and around infected follicles and in pseudogranules.
- Differentials include other infectious or foreign body granulomata, sterile panniculitis, neoplasia.

Treatment
- Surgical excision or debulking in conjunction with long-term systemic antifungal therapy:
  - No licensed products available; off-label use of human fluconazole, either initial dose of 14 mg/kg by mouth followed by 5 mg/kg twice daily by mouth, or 10 mg/kg by mouth once daily, for extended period.
  - Maybe cost-prohibitive; generic drugs less expensive than brand names.
- Prognosis guarded; full resolution difficult to achieve.

Fungal mycetoma

Clinical features
- Chronic subcutaneous infection where fungi are present in tissues as granules or grains.
- Cause:
  - Eumycotic mycetoma: soil-living species *Curvularia geniculata,* (pigmented grains) *Pseudallescheria boydii* (non-pigmented grains).

- Signs:
  - Chronic subcutaneous nodules, usually solitary, often ulcerated with draining tracts and tissue granules or grains in discharge (Figure 5.13).
  - Lesions may involve underlying tissues including bone.

Diagnosis
- Clinical signs.
- Stained smears of exudate or needle aspirate.
- Fungal culture of tissue grains.
- Biopsy for histopathology and fungal culture:
  - Nodular to diffuse, granulomatous to pyogranulomatous dermatitis, and panniculitis with fungal elements in grains or granules, which may or may not be pigmented.
- Differentials: other infectious granulomata, foreign body granulomata, neoplasia.

Treatment
- Wide surgical excision offers the best chance of cure.
- Systemic treatment with off-label human antifungals, ideally on the basis of susceptibility testing of isolate; choices include fluconazole, (see dosage above), itraconazole (stability issues with compounded preparations), voriconazole (often cost-prohibitive), and amphotericin B (risk of nephrotoxicity).

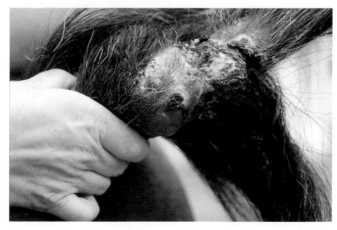

Figure 5.13 Fungal mycetoma affecting the tail; caused by soil-living organisms.

- Systemic iodides:
  - Limited efficacy, now considered substandard method of treating fungal diseases in horses.
- Prognosis is guarded; medical therapy often unsuccessful.

Phaeohyphomycosis (chromomycosis)

Clinical features
- Rare lesions caused by wound contamination with saprophytic fungi that form pigmented hyphal elements, but not tissue grains.
- Causes include *Drechslera spicifera*, *Alternaria* spp., *Cladosporium* spp., and others.
- Signs:
  - Firm, non-painful nodules, usually with normal overlying skin and hair.
  - Occasionally alopecia, hyperpigmented, ulcerated, draining lesions.
  - Mostly multiple lesions, affecting any part of body.
- Differentials include other infectious granulomata, foreign body granulomata, sterile granulomata, neoplasia.

Diagnosis
- Smears of exudate or aspirates:
  - Pyogranulomatous inflammation with fungal elements, septate hyphae, but no tissue grains.
- Biopsy for histopathology and fungal culture at 25–35 °C:
  - Nodular to diffuse, granulomatous to pyogranulomatous inflammation with numerous pigmented septate fungal hyphae and yeast forms, but tissue grains absent.

Treatment
- Wide surgical excision; may be curative.
- Concomitant use or sole use of (off-label) systemic fluconazole (10 mg/kg once daily or loading dose of 14 mg/kg by mouth followed by 5 mg/kg twice daily) for extended period.
- Prognosis guarded; poor response to medical therapy.

Sporotrichosis

Clinical features
- Rare disease in Europe, more common in southern USA; usually occurs through wound contamination.

- Usually only one horse in a herd affected.
- Risk of zoonotic spread to humans.
- Cause:
  - *Sporothrix schenckii*, ubiquitous saprophytic fungus.
- Signs:
  - Hard, subcutaneous nodules often on distal limbs, which ulcerate and produce creamy pus.
  - Draining lymphatics often thickened and enlarged (corded).
  - Chronic ulcerated lesions may develop granulation tissue.

Diagnosis
- Cytological examination of smears or exudate, or aspirates; fungal culture of material from a deep tract:
  - Suppurative pyogranulomatous inflammation; organism is hard to find.
- Biopsy for histopathological examination and fungal culture at 30 °C:
  - Nodular to diffuse, pyogranulomatous to granulomatous dermatitis and panniculitis.
  - Pleomorphic yeast organisms with refractile cell wall may be sparse, occasionally numerous.
  - Direct immunofluorescence to demonstration *Sporothrix* antigen.
- Differentials: infectious mycetomata, foreign body granulomata, exuberant granulation tissue, neoplasia.

Treatment
- Fluconazole (10 mg/kg once daily or loading dose of 14 mg/kg by mouth followed by 5 mg/kg twice daily) for extended period.
- Systemic iodides:
  - Limited efficacy, now considered substandard method of treating fungal diseases in horses.

Other subcutaneous and deep mycotic infections

A number of other saprophytes and fungus-like organisms may cause cutaneous lesions in horses in certain geographical locations. Conditions are typically characterised by ulcerated nodules and draining tracts. Deep fungal infections cause systemic disease that may also disseminate to the skin.

- Pythiosis, caused by *Pythium insidiosum*, an aquatic fungus-like organism, occurs in tropical and subtropical regions.

- Zygomycosis, caused by saprophytes including *Rhizopus*, *Mucor*, *Absidia*, *Conidiobolus*, and *Basidiobolus* occurs in tropical and subtropical regions, particularly along the Gulf of Mexico.
- Rhinosporidiosis, caused by *Rhinosporidium*, is endemic in India and Sri Lanka, sporadic in Africa, Europe, and the Americas.
- Systemic mycoses that include blastomycosis, coccidiomycosis, and cryptococcosis, caused by saprophytic yeast-like fungal organisms, are rare and, apart from very occasional cases of cryptococcosis, not seen in Europe.

PARASITIC CONDITIONS

Hypodermiasis (warbles)

Clinical features
- Eradicated from the UK, but might occur in imported horses; still found in many countries in the northern hemisphere.
- Cause:
  - Infestation by larvae of warble flies, *Hypoderma bovis*, *H. lineatum*.
- Cattle are primary hosts.
- Seasonal incidence around spring.
- Signs:
  - Subcutaneous nodules and cysts over dorsum.
  - Opening or breathing pore frequently develops.
  - Sometimes painful.
  - Anaphylaxis reported following death or rupture of larvae.

Diagnosis
- History and clinical signs, animal imported to the UK; contact with cattle in other countries.
- Demonstration of larvae.
- Differentials: infectious granulomata, cysts, eosinophilic granuloma, neoplasia.

Treatment
- Gentle enlargement of pore and extraction of larvae.
- Surgical excision of entire nodule.
- Allow natural extrusion of larva.
- Prevention:

- Fly control.
- Worming with avermectins should prevent larval migration and development.

Parafilariasis

See Chapter 4.

Filariasis

Clinical features
- Nodular cutaneous lesions associated with the nematode, *Onchocerca boehmi*, have been reported in horses in Europe and the Middle East; lifecycle of this helminth is uncertain.
- Lesions are non-painful, well circumscribed, and firm.

Diagnosis
- Histopathological examination of biopsy material reveals fragments of larval nematodes.

Treatment
- Avermectins (ivermectin (Bimectin Horse Oral Paste, Bimeda; Animec Oral Paste for Horses, Chanelle Pharma; Eqvalan Oral Paste for Horses, Boehringer Ingelheim Animal Health UK; Vectin Horse Oral Paste, MSD Animal Health UK; Eraquell Oral Paste, Virbac; Noromectin, Norbrook Laboratories) 200 µg/kg or moxidectin (Equest Oral Gel for Horses and Ponies, Zoetis UK) 400 µg/kg,), two oral doses at 3-week intervals should secure resolution of lesions, with adjunctive use of glucocorticoids as needed.

Demodicosis

Clinical features
- Rare.
- Cause:
  - Excessive numbers of commensal mites, *Demodex equi* or *D. caballi*, in situations of immune suppression.
- Signs:
  - Alopecia, scaling, and variable pyoderma (Figure 5.14).
  - Nodular form, less common.

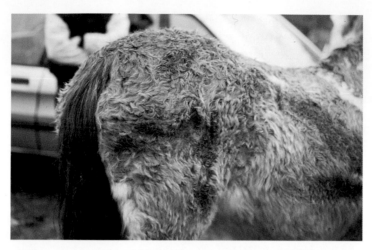

Figure 5.14 Demodicosis and folliculitis associated with alopecia, erythema, and excoriation in a 23-year-old pony; appearance suggestive of underlying pituitary pars intermedia dysfunction (PPID).

Diagnosis
- History and clinical signs; concurrent disease or immunosuppressive therapy such as glucocorticoids.
- Demonstration of mites in skin scrapings or material expressed from nodules.
- Differentials: infectious granulomata, hypodermiasis, cysts, eosinophilic granuloma, neoplasia.

Treatment
- Treat underlying disease, discontinue glucocorticoid therapy; may result in spontaneous regression.
- Oral avermectins may be effective.
- Amitraz may cause death in horses and is absolutely contraindicated.
- Prognosis is fair to guarded, depending on underlying factors.

Leishmaniasis

Clinical features
- In regions where *Leishmania* parasites are endemic, horses and donkeys may become infected.
- Equids are resistant to infection, and clinical disease, when it occurs, is mild.

- Presence of seroconversion is variable, depending upon endemicity and availability of hosts for sand fly (*Phlebotomus* spp.) feeding.
- Species associated with cutaneous infection in equidae:
  - *Leishmania braziliensis*, *L. infantum*, and *L. martiniquensis* (previously known as *L. siamensis*).
- Promastigotes introduced when sand flies feed parasitise macrophages, forming amastigotes with subsequent multiplication.
- Signs:
  - Single or multiple papules or nodules 5–20 mm diameter at sites of sand fly feeding; head, neck, pinnae, axillae, inguinal regions; nodules may ulcerate.
  - Visceral signs not seen.

Diagnosis
- Identification of parasitic amastigotes in macrophages in skin biopsies, lymph node aspirates, peripheral blood.
- Serology, but tests require standardisation and may give false-positive and false-negative results.
- Confirmation of current infection and identification of species by PCR.
- Differentials: eosinophilic granuloma, infectious granulomata, insect bites, urticaria, erythema multiforme.

Treatment
- Disease is self-limiting, resolution usually in 3–4 or up to 6 months, associated with cell-mediated immunity.
- Surgical removal of nodules.
- Prevention:
  - Avoidance of insect vector by stabling at night, use of insect repellents and insecticides.

IMMUNE-MEDIATED CONDITIONS

Urticaria and angio-oedema

Clinical features
- Urticaria (hives): papules, wheals, plaques, varying in extent, which pit on pressure and are transient (Figure 5.15).
- Lesions especially on neck and trunk, but can affect any part of the body.
- Angio-oedema: large oedematous swellings (Figure 5.16), often in dependent areas; may ooze serous fluid.

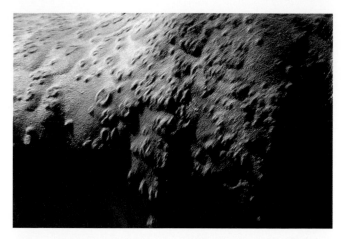

Figure 5.15 Urticaria. Multiple raised papules, plaques, and annular lesions on the trunk and shoulder region.

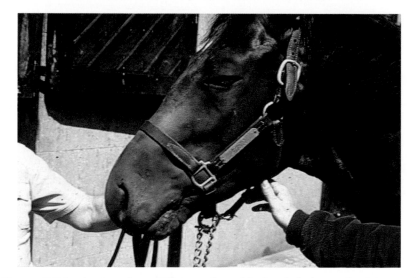

Figure 5.16 Angio-oedema. Diffuse swelling of the head of a horse after injection of a non-steroidal anti-inflammatory drug. Source: Pilsworth and Knottenbelt (2007), figure 4, p. 369. Reproduced with permission of Equine Veterinary Education.

- Results from mast cell degranulation due to type I hypersensitivity reactions or mechanical mechanisms.
- Individual lesions often transient, but new lesions may develop.
- Pruritus may be present.
- Causes:
  - Hypersensitivity disorders (see atopic dermatitis in Chapter 2), physical factors (pressure, exercise, heat/cold, light), topical and systemic

drugs, chemicals (including soaps, leather conditioners), insect bites, infections (e.g. dermatophytosis), vaccines, food stuffs.

Diagnosis
- History, signs; lesions pit on application of digital pressure.
- Careful history to identify potential causal factors.
- Restriction/elimination tests and provocative challenge:
  - Maintain fully outdoors/indoors.
  - Change bedding.
  - Elimination diet of exclusively grass (grass nuts, hay, haylage).
  - Change detergents, change products used on leather, and tack items.
- Allergen-specific IgE testing in cases where other causes ruled out and clinical diagnosis of atopic dermatitis reached.
- Biopsy. Histopathology non-diagnostic, with non-specific findings of oedema and variable superficial perivascular dermatitis, but may help with rule-outs.
- Differentials include early dermatophytosis, erythema multiforme, amyloidosis.

Treatment
- Identify and eliminate causes.
  - In cases of suspected adverse drug reactions, further exposure or challenge is contraindicated.
- Symptomatic treatment:
  - Prednisolone 0.5–1 mg/kg once daily by mouth until control is achieved, then reduce to lowest alternate-day regimen. Alternatively, dexamethasone short-acting injection (Dexa-Ject, Bimeda; Duphacort Q, Zoetis; Dexadreson, MSD Animal Health, Colvasone, Norbrook Laboratories; Rapidexon, Dechra) 0.01–0.02 mg/kg intramuscularly as a loading dose followed by oral prednisolone or use of dexamethasone tablets (Dexacortone, Dechra Veterinary Products, off-label use) 0.02–0.1 mg/kg by mouth every 48–72 hours.
  - Antihistamines: none is licensed for veterinary use, but the following tablets may be useful alone or as steroid-sparing agents.
    - Hydroxyzine (Atarax, Pfizer) 0.5–2 mg/kg twice or three times daily.
    - Chlorphenamine, formerly chlorpheniramine, (Piriton, Allercalm, Hayleve) 0.25–0.5 mg/kg twice or three times daily.
    - Diphenhydramine (Nytol capsules) 1–2 mg/kg twice or three times daily.

- ○ Alimemazine, formerly trimeprazine, (Zentiva) 1–2 mg/kg twice or three times daily.
  - ○ Cetirizine (Zyrtec) 0.2–0.4 mg/kg twice daily.
- Prognosis for urticaria is usually good; many cases may only suffer one episode but, where signs persist or are recurrent over 3–6 weeks, further investigation is warranted; for angio-oedema, prognosis is variable depending on severity, location, and presence of other signs of anaphylaxis.

Dermatographism

Clinical features
- Degranulation of cutaneous mast cells caused by application of pressure.
- Associated with type 1 hypersensitivity conditions.
- Signs: oedematous, linear wheals at sites of application of pressure such as tack, harness.

Diagnosis
- History, characteristic clinical signs.
- Confirm by application of pressure to the skin with blunt object (Figure 5.17).
- Investigate underlying causes of urticaria.

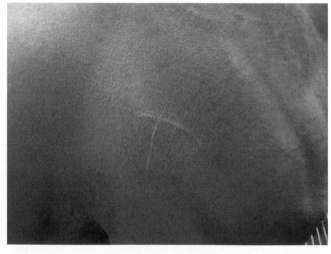

Figure 5.17 Linear urticarial wheals in a cruciform shape on the shoulder of an atopic horse which resulted from application of pressure by a capped ballpoint pen.

Treatment
- Identify and eliminate underlying causes.
- Symptomatic treatment as above.

Cutaneous amyloidosis

Clinical features
- Rare cause of skin disease, usually with concurrent upper respiratory signs; skin not usually involved in cases of systemic amyloidosis.
- Accumulations of fibrillar deposits of immunoglobulin light chains.
- Unknown triggering factors.
- Signs:
  - Multiple papules, nodules, plaques, firm and well-circumscribed, non-painful, commonly affecting head (Figure 5.18), neck, shoulders, and pectoral regions; variable regional lymphadenopathy.
  - Onset may be rapid and resemble urticaria; usually chronic, progressive course.
  - Accompanying or preceded by upper respiratory tract signs.

Diagnosis
- Needle aspirates, skin biopsy for definitive diagnosis.
- Histopathology confirms presence of extracellular amyloid deposits, granulomatous dermatitis and panniculitis with multinucleate histiocytic giant cells.
- Differentials: eosinophilic granuloma, cutaneous lymphoma, other neoplasms.

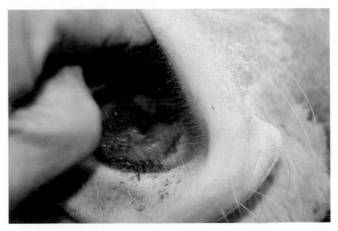

Figure 5.18   Cutaneous amyloidosis. Raised, firm plaque affecting the mucocutaneous junctional region of the external naris. Source: Courtesy of Kieran O'Brien.

Treatment
- No proven effective treatment, but may see temporary amelioration with glucocorticoids or progestagens.

NEOPLASIA

Sarcoid

Clinical features
- The most common equine neoplasm.
- No age or sex predisposition, but genetic predisposition associated with certain haplotypes of leucocyte antigen; polygenic trait with >20% heritability reported in a Swiss breed.
- Strong association with bovine papilloma virus (BPV)-1 or less frequently BPV-2.
- Insect vectors likely as BPV detected in biting flies from farms with affected horses.
- May be single or multiple.
- Tend to occur on sparsely haired areas, particularly head, inguinal regions, ventrum.
- Often only slowly progressive, but trauma may result in progression of lesions.
- Six clinical forms described:
  - Occult: flat, alopecic lesions, mild surface scaling, minimal skin thickening (Figure 5.19).
  - Verrucose: wart-like, alopecic, thickened skin, surface hyperkeratosis (Figure 5.20).
  - Nodular: overlying skin intact, may be moveable over lesion or attached and infiltrated (Figure 5.21).
  - Fibroblastic: fleshy, ulcerated, may be pedunculated or sessile and broad-based with dermal or subdermal extensions (Figure 5.22).
  - Mixed.
  - Malevolent/malignant: invasive, rapidly proliferative, with lymphatic spread (Figure 5.23).

Diagnosis
- Physical appearance, location.
- Biopsy and histopathology required for confirmation:

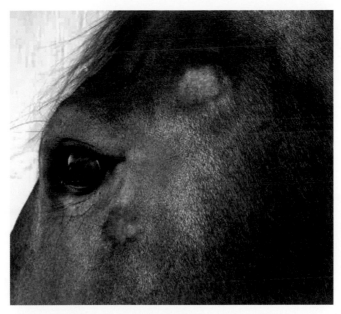

Figure 5.19 Occult (flat) sarcoids. Two annular areas of alopecia with mild surface scaling on the face.

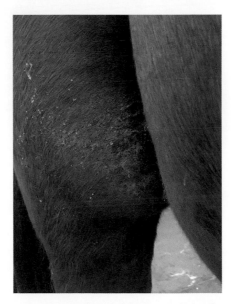

Figure 5.20 Verrucose sarcoid. Plaque of thickened skin with surface hyperkeratosis and warty appearance affecting the gluteal region of an 11-year-old horse; lesion progressed over months to palpable nodules.

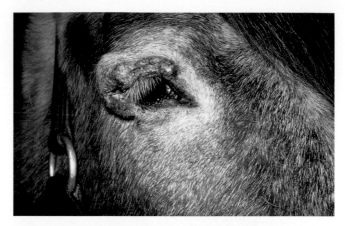

Figure 5.21   Nodular sarcoids affecting the periocular region. Source: Courtesy of K.C. Barnett.

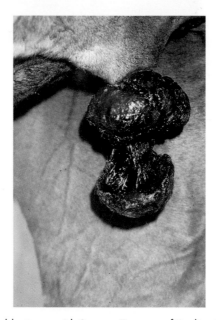

Figure 5.22   Fibroblastic sarcoid. Source: Courtesy of Pauline Williams.

- Although there is a risk of exacerbation, this is difficult to quantify and should not preclude making a proper diagnosis so that optimal treatment can be instituted.
- Differentials:
  - Occult: mild repeated trauma/rubs, dermatophytosis, dermatophilosis, folliculitis, linear keratosis, alopecia areata, pemphigus foliaceous, sarcoidosis.

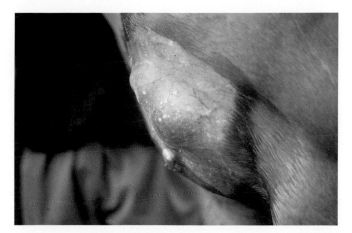

Figure 5.23 Malevolent/malignant sarcoid. Source: Courtesy of Andrew Browning.

- Verrucose: papillomatosis, chronic trauma with hyperkeratosis and lichenification, sarcoidosis, squamous cell carcinoma.
- Nodular: eosinophilic granuloma, fibroma/fibrosarcoma, melanoma, Schwannoma, lymphosarcoma, cysts.
- Fibroblastic: exuberant granulation tissue, bacterial/fungal granulomata, habronemiasis, squamous cell carcinoma, fibrosarcoma.
- Malevolent: lymphangitis, cellulitis.

Treatment
- There is no single, entirely reliable treatment and all cases should be handled on an individual basis, after careful assessment, taking specialist advice where appropriate.
- Benign neglect:
  - May be appropriate to monitor small lesions in areas not interfering with tack.
  - Any signs of growth or change should initiate intervention.
  - Early treatment of small lesions in young horses carries a better prognosis.
- Surgical removal:
  - Sharp excision: not recommended, carries high risk of seeding of tumour cells and recurrence.
  - Cryotherapy, with or without prior debulking; high recurrence rates.
  - Laser surgery excision: surgical option of choice, with >80% cure rate after first treatment, >70% cure rate after second procedures.
- Radiation: brachytherapy using implanted radioisotopes (gold[198], iridium[192]); requires specialist nursing in designated radiation facilities. Success rates of 81–100% reported for iridium brachytherapy.

- Intralesional therapy:
  - Cytotoxic agents (unlicensed use):
    - Mitomycin (0.04% mitomycin C) injections for nodular or fibroblastic lesions, repeated every 8 weeks; 96% overall cure rate after range of 1–5 injections reported, higher for periocular lesions.
    - Cisplatin emulsion in oil; requires extreme care in preparation, handling, and administration. Cure rates of 87–97% described.
  - Immunomodulation (unlicensed use):
    - BCG (bacillus Calmette-Guérin) vaccine is most effective for periocular sarcoids, may exacerbate lesions elsewhere; hypersensitivity reactions may occur and concurrent administration of antihistamines and, or, glucocorticoids is suggested.
- Topical therapy
  - Immunomodulation;
    - Imiquimod 5% cream (Aldara, Meda Pharmaceuticals) is a local immunostimulant licensed for treatment of genital warts and certain skin cancers in humans; has been shown to be effective in equine sarcoid (off-label use), with 80% of cases showing >75% reduction and 60% cured in 8–32 weeks. Thin film of cream is applied to the lesions three times weekly, removed by gentle washing after 6-10 hours to limit inflammation. Can be used on all types of sarcoid at all anatomical sites, applied by owners; improved cure rate with extended periods of treatment.
  - Cytotoxic agents:
    - Liverpool sarcoid cream (AW4-LUDES cream) is a compounded, unlicensed product containing antimitotics and cytotoxics including arsenic trioxide, podophyllin, and 5-fluoruracil; is hazardous and is dispensed for application by veterinarians to tumours daily or every other day until resolution; it causes significant inflammation, and swelling and pain in some cases.
    - Blood root ointments (Xxterra, Vetline, Fort Collins USA; Sarcoff, Forum Animal Health, Bexhill UK; Newmarket Bloodroot Ointment, Newmarket Premixes, Hatfield UK) containing alkaloid extracts from the rhizome of *Sanguinaria canadensis* plants have been shown to be of benefit in management of equine sarcoids; unlicensed products, marketed as adjuncts to treatment of sarcoids. May cause significant inflammation and contraindicated for use on the face.
- Prognosis is poorer in cases that have had previous treatments.
- Preventive measures to include insect control on premises where there are affected animals.

Squamous cell carcinoma

Clinical features

- Second most common equine tumour, accounting for 20% of all tumour cases; most common periocular and periadnexal tumour.
- Mean age incidence of 12 years; no breed predilection but males over-represented because of genital lesions.
- Associated with chronic exposure to ultraviolet light of unpigmented, poorly haired skin.
- Penile and preputial lesions following malignant transformation of papillomatous lesions associated with papillomavirus EcPV-2.
- Signs:
  - Mucocutaneous junctions of head (Figure 5.24) and external genitalia (Figure 5.25) are common sites.
  - Lesions usually proliferative with secondary ulceration; sometimes primarily erosive.
  - May present as chronic, non-healing ulcer.
  - Haemorrhage and secondary infection may occur.

Diagnosis

- History and clinical signs.
- Histopathological examination of excised or biopsied tissue for confirmation.
- Differentials: habronemiasis, exuberant granulation tissue, fibroblastic sarcoid, other neoplasms.

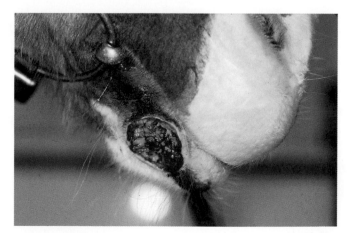

Figure 5.24 Squamous cell carcinoma. Ulcerated mass on the non-pigmented lower lip of a 25-year-old horse. Regional lymphadenopathy was also present. Source: Courtesy of M.J. Brearley.

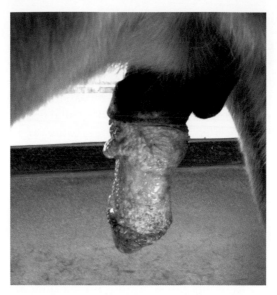

Figure 5.25 Penile squamous cell carcinoma. Nodules, together with multiple papillomata, on shaft of penis due to neoplastic transformation of genital papillomata associated with EcPV-2 infection.

Treatment
- Wide surgical excision, cryosurgery, laser surgery.
- Radiotherapy: brachytherapy with radioisotopes including gold[198] and iridium[192].
- Cytotoxic chemotherapy:
  - Intralesional cisplatin injections
  - Topical 5-fluorouracil (off-label use of human product) applied daily.
- Intralesional BCG (off-label use of human product) reported to be beneficial.
- Prognosis:
  - Locally aggressive and may spread to local lymph nodes; distant metastasis possible.
  - Penile and preputial lesions tend to be more aggressive and less amenable to non-surgical management.

Melanocytic tumours

Melanocytic nevi

Clinical features
- Pigmented cutaneous nodules, usually solitary, occurring at a variety of sites.
- Seen in young horses of any colour.
- Lesion is at dermo-epidermal junction.

Diagnosis
- History and clinical signs.
- Confirmation by examination of smears of final needle aspirates, biopsy for histopathology.
- Differentials: melanoma; melanomatosis.

Treatment
- Surgical excision is curative.

Melanoma, Malignant Melanoma and Melanomatosis

Clinical features
- Common neoplasm of grey and white-coated horses; almost ubiquitous in older animals. Very low prevalence in non-grey animals. No sex predilection.
- Single or multiple discreet lesions (melanoma) or coalescing lesions (melanomatosis); can be found in skin and internal organs.
- Can be multifocal with distant dissemination (malignant melanoma).
- Signs:
  - Heavily pigmented firm nodules or masses in deep dermis.
  - Predilection for tail, perineum, vulva (Figure 5.26), dorsal prepuce, commissures of lips, parotid salivary gland; also occur at other external and many internal locations.

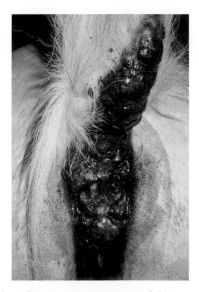

Figure 5.26 Multiple melanocytic tumours around the anus, vulva, and ventral tail base of a mare with melanoma.

- Sometimes ulcerative with a black discharge.
- Lymphadenopathy of local drainage lymph nodes.
- Pelvic masses may interfere with defaecation and involve neural and vascular tissues resulting in various clinical signs.
- Parotid lesions may impinge on upper airway and movement of neck.

Diagnosis
- History and clinical signs.
- Confirmation by examination of smears of final needle aspirates, biopsy for histopathology.
- Differentials: melanocytic nevus.

Treatment
- Surgical excision whilst lesions are small. No evidence of activation of disease.
- Laser surgery with postoperative wound management; associated with good recovery rate and low recurrence.
- Intralesional cisplatin injections or implantation of beads (unlicensed) reported to be effective in small lesions and as an adjunct to surgery where complete excision is not possible.
- Cimetidine (off-label use) has failed to give consistent benefit.
- Long-term prognosis is guarded to poor in long-standing cases. However, early surgical removal of lesions can prevent disease progression and reduced incidence of distant metastases.

Anaplastic malignant melanoma

Clinical features
- Uncommon tumour of older horses of any coat colour.
- Often metastasised by time of diagnosis.
- Signs:
  - Variably pigmented masses.
  - Predilection site of tail and tail head (Figure 5.27).

Diagnosis
- History and clinical signs.
- Biopsy for histopathological examination.
- Differential diagnosis: melanoma/melanomatosis; melanocytic nevus; sarcoid; squamous cell carcinoma; fibroma/fibrosarcoma.

Treatment
- As for melanoma above, but prognosis is poor.

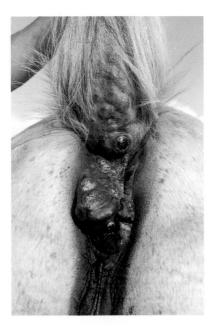

Figure 5.27 Amelanotic melanomas affecting the perineum and ventral tail base.

Other cutaneous neoplasms

Mastocytoma (mast cell tumour, mastocytosis)

Clinical features
- Uncommon, usually benign tumours.
- No breed predilection; Thoroughbreds may be under-represented.
- Age range 1–25 years, average 9.5 years; males predisposed.
- Signs:
  - Usually solitary, raised, firm, well-demarcated nodules or masses (Figure 5.28).
  - Overlying skin may be normal, alopecic, hyperpigmented, or ulcerated.
  - Occasionally, areas become fluctuant and discharge caseous material.
  - Most commonly affect head, particularly muzzle, also neck, trunk, and limbs.
  - Rarely, multiple widespread lesions occur in foals, with similarities to human urticaria pigmentosa.

Diagnosis
- Cytological examination of fine needle aspirates demonstrates presence of mast cells.
- Histopathological examination of biopsies to confirm. Differentiation from other round cell tumours may be difficult.

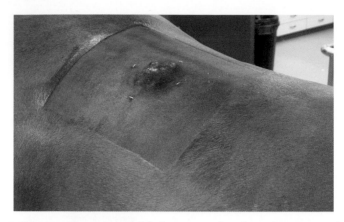

Figure 5.28 Mastocytoma. Multilobular mass with surface ulceration on the dorsal trunk; staples inserted prior to laser removal to ensure adequate surgical margins. Source: Courtesy of Richard Payne.

Treatment
- Complete surgical excision is curative; spontaneous remission may occur after incomplete excision or biopsy.
- Sublesional injections of glucocorticoid, 5–10 mg of triamcinolone acetonide (not licensed for veterinary use in the UK) or 10–20 mg methylprednisolone acetate (Depo-Medrone V suspension for injection, Zoetis UK).
- Cryosurgery or radiotherapy may be effective.
- Occasional horses develop new lesions in different sites over years.
- Widespread metastasis not reported; rarely involvement of local lymph nodes reported. Skin involvement in primary internal organ disease may occur very rarely.

Fibroma/fibrosarcoma

Clinical features
- Rare neoplasms of the skin.
- Adult to aged horses, no breed or sex predilection.
- Signs:
  - Usually solitary dermal to subcutaneous lesions.
  - Periocular region, neck, limbs, sometimes trunk.
  - Benign lesions are firm to soft, well-circumscribed, with overlying skin usually normal.
  - Malignant lesions are poorly demarcated, firm to fleshy, infiltrative subcutaneous masses, frequently ulcerated and secondarily infected.

Diagnosis
- Cytological examination of fine needle aspirates may demonstrate spindle-shaped cells, which may be atypical in malignant form.
- Confirmation by histopathological examination of excised tissue or biopsy; malignant tumours show more frequent mitoses and cellular atypia; both forms are positive for vimentin.
- Differentials: sarcoid, other skin tumours.

Treatment
- Surgical excision with wide margins usually curative for benign disease, but recurrence is common with fibrosarcomas.
- Other options include:
  - Radiotherapy with gold[198] or iridium[192].
  - Intralesional cytotoxic agents.
  - Topical 5-fluoruracil application (off-label use).
- Prognosis for benign lesions is good; although malignant lesions often recur, distant metastasis is very rare.

Schwannoma (Peripheral nerve sheath tumour)

Clinical features
- Rare neoplasms arising from perineural cells.
- Adult horses, no breed or sex predisposition.
- Solitary, firm nodules, overlying skin and hair coat normal; may become multilobulated.
- No site predilection.

Diagnosis
- Histopathological examination of biopsy or excised tissue.
- Differentials: sarcoid, fibroma, fibrosarcoma, other skin neoplasms.

Treatment
- Surgical excision but may recur.
- Other options include:
  - Radiotherapy with gold[198] or iridium[192].
  - Intralesional cytotoxic agents.
- Prognosis fair to guarded; recurrence rate for periocular lesions is 50%.

Lipoma

Clinical features
- Rare, benign tumour arising from subcutaneous lipocytes.
- Young adult horses, no sex or breed predisposition.
- Signs:
  - Solitary, well-circumscribed, soft to fleshy, variable sized subcutaneous masses.
  - Usually slow-growing, overlying skin normal.
  - Most commonly on trunk and proximal limbs.
  - Sometimes locally infiltrative.

Diagnosis
- Cytological examination of fine needle aspirates.
- Histopathological confirmation of biopsy or excised tissue.

Treatment
- Surgical excision.
- Leave and monitor.
- Prognosis good apart from the very rare cases of malignant liposarcoma.

Cutaneous lymphoma (Lymphosarcoma)

Clinical features
- Rare neoplasm of adult to aged horses.
- No sex or breed predilection.
- Two forms described:
  - Epitheliotropic lymphoma of T-lymphocyte origin.
  - Non-epitheliotropic lymphoma involving skin and subcutis, may be B-cell or T-cell origin.
- Signs:
  - Non-epitheliotropic:
    - Cutaneous lesions usually multiple and widespread, firm, well-circumscribed papules and nodules to masses, dermal to subcutaneous.
    - Head, neck, and proximal limbs typically involved.
    - Usually associated with internal organ involvement (multicentric disease) and associated clinical signs of lymphadenopathy, weight loss, lethargy.

- o Some horses with lymphohistiocytic phenotype have only skin lesions, which may wax and wane for months to years (Figure 5.29) before progressing to systemic involvement (primary cutaneous disease).
- – Epitheliotropic:
  - o Multifocal to generalised exfoliative dermatitis with alopecia, scaling, and crusting.
  - o May have focal areas of nodules or ulceration.
  - o Maybe pruritic and may show erythroderma.

Diagnosis
- Cytological examination of fine needle aspirates.
- Confirmation by histopathological examination of skin biopsies.
- Immunohistochemistry to determine cell line; most cases are T-cell in origin.
- Differentials: eosinophilic granuloma, sterile panniculitis, sarcoid, fibroma, mastocytoma, melanoma, squamous cell carcinoma, amyloidosis.

Treatment
- Prognosis for horses with epitheliotropic disease and those with concurrent systemic disease is grave; death or euthanasia usually ensues within weeks to months.

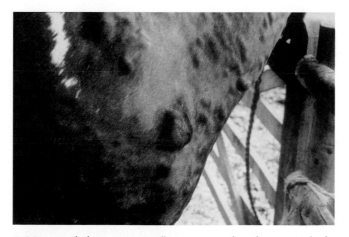

Figure 5.29 Lymphohistiocytic T-cell cutaneous lymphoma. Multiple nodules, plaques, and masses on the neck and shoulder of a 15-year-old horse with an 11-year history of waxing and waning disease. Source: Littlewood et al. (1995), figure 1, p.106. Reproduced with permission of Veterinary Dermatology.

- Horses with primary cutaneous lymphoma have shown extended survival with various treatments including:
  - Sublesional injections of depot glucocorticoids.
  - Oral glucocorticoids, initially daily then low-dose alternate-day therapy.
  - Oral progestogens.

MISCELLANEOUS CAUSES

Bites and stings

Clinical features
- Nettles, wasps, bees, biting flies, spiders, and snakes.
- Signs vary according to agent, amount of venom injected, host factors.
- Signs:
  - Papules, wheals, plaques, diffuse swelling (Figure 5.30).
  - Variable pain and pruritus.
  - Anaphylaxis.
  - Necrosis and sloughing.

Diagnosis
- History and clinical signs; acute onset.
- Differentials: other causes of urticaria; eosinophilic granuloma, unilateral papular dermatosis, haematomata, abscesses, cysts; poisoning.

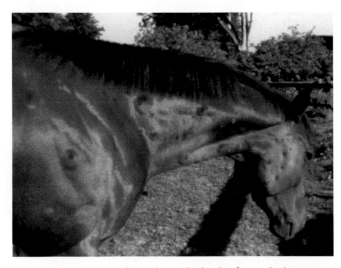

Figure 5.30 Multiple urticarial papules and wheals after multiple mosquito bites.

Treatment
- Leave alone.
- Symptomatic treatment with glucocorticoids, antihistamines.
- Other supportive therapy as indicated.
- Insect repellents.
- Prognosis varies according to source of bite or sting and host factors.

Eosinophilic granuloma

Clinical features
- Common skin conditions of horses of any age, sex, breed.
- Occurs mostly in spring and summer.
- Lesions may regress spontaneously, but recurrence is common; mineralised lesions are often persistent.
- Cause:
  - Uncertain, likely multifactorial, but hypersensitivity to insect bites implicated; maybe seen in atopic animals.
- Collagen lysis/necrosis is not a feature; synonyms 'collagenolytic granuloma' and 'collagen necrosis' are misnomers.
- Signs:
  - Single or multiple dermal papules, nodules, variable diameter (Figure 5.31).
  - Often in saddle areas, but also neck, trunk, flank, but may occur anywhere.

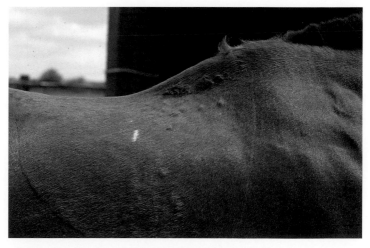

Figure 5.31   Papular lesions of eosinophilic granuloma.

- Well-circumscribed, firm, non-alopecic, usually non-painful and non-pruritic.
- Overlying skin surface and hair usually normal unless traumatised.
- Mineralisation in chronic lesions; extrusion of calcified material may be seen as a central whitish pore.

Diagnosis

- History and clinical signs; may show signs of concurrent hypersensitivity disorders, which should be investigated as appropriate.
- Stained smears of needle aspirates, but aspirates may yield little material.
- Skin biopsy for histopathological examination:
  - Nodular to diffuse eosinophilic, granulomatous dermatitis, collagen flame figures (fibres partially or totally surrounded by amorphous to granular eosinophilic material in variable configurations; fibres may appear fuzzy due to coating with eosinophilic material, but are not degenerate), foci of eosinophilic folliculitis or furunculosis may be present; dystrophic mineralisation of older lesions.
- Differentials: habronemiasis, injection site reactions, arthropod bites, infectious granulomata, mast cell tumours.

Treatment

- Leave alone; modify padding for lesions localised to saddle region.
- Surgical excision of solitary or low numbers of lesions.
- Glucocorticoids: systemic, intralesional or sublesional injections of long-acting formulations:
  - Prednisolone 1–2 mg/kg once daily by mouth for 2–3 weeks, then alternate-day dosing and taper according to clinical response.
  - Dexamethasone tablets (not licensed for veterinary use in the UK) 0.1 mg/kg by mouth once every 24 hours for 2–3 weeks.
  - Triamcinolone acetonide (not licensed for veterinary use in the UK) intra- or sublesional injection, 3–5 mg per lesions. No more than 20 mg per horse. Repeat after 2 weeks if necessary.
  - Dexamethasone suspension for injection (Dexafort, MSD Animal Health) could be considered as an alternative; dose equivalent would be 0.6–1 mg per lesion; licensed for doses of 1 ml (4 mg)/kg bodyweight.
  - Methylprednisolone acetate (Depo-Medrone V suspension for injection, Zoetis UK) intra- or sublesional injection, 5–10 mg per lesion; licensed for doses of 80–400 mg in synovial structures, 200 mg per horse for intramuscular use.

- Prognosis fair to guarded:
  - Lesions often recur, permanent remission is unlikely.
  - Glucocorticoids less effective for chronic, mineralised lesions.
  - Risk of laminitis after administration of depot steroid preparations.

Unilateral papular dermatosis

Clinical features
- Uncommon to rare.
- Often seasonal, spring and summer.
- Cause thought to be reaction to insect or arthropod bites.
- Signs:
  - Multiple papules and nodules limited to one side of body, usually thorax, but also neck and trunk.
  - Firm, elevated, well-circumscribed, may become crusted; pruritus and pain absent.

Diagnosis
- Clinical presentation, confirmation by needle aspirates, skin biopsy:
  - Eosinophilic folliculitis and furunculosis, sometimes with collagen flame figures; special stains and cultures negative.
- Differentials: eosinophilic granuloma, staphylococcal folliculitis/furunculosis, dermatophytosis, calcinosis circumscripta, neoplasia.

Treatment
- Leave alone.
- Glucocorticoids systemically:
  - Prednisolone 1–2 mg/kg once daily by mouth for 2–3 weeks, then alternate-day dosing and taper according to clinical response.
  - Dexamethasone tablets (Dexacortone, Dechra Veterinary Products, off-label use) 0.1 mg/kg by mouth once daily for 2–3 weeks.
- Prognosis usually good:
  - Some cases spontaneously resolve after a few weeks or months.
  - Response to glucocorticoids is usually rapid.
  - Sometimes recurs in subsequent years.
- Insect control, repellents for prophylaxis.

Axillary nodular necrosis

Clinical features
- Rare condition of mature horses.
- Both working and non-working animals.

- Only one of a group affected.
- Cause is unknown.
- Signs:
  - Usually unilateral, single, or multiple lesions.
  - Round, firm, well-circumscribed, non-alopecic, non-painful, non-pruritic, subcutaneous nodules in the axilla or girth regions.
  - Overlying skin and hair usually normal; occasional lesions may ulcerate.

Diagnosis
- Clinical presentation.
- Smears of aspirates, skin biopsies:
  - Eosinophilic granulomatous inflammation, nodular to diffuse dermatitis and panniculitis, focal necrosis; vasculopathic changes present, but may need multiple sections to identify.
- Differential: infectious or sterile granulomata, cysts, neoplasia.

Treatment
- Leave alone.
- Surgical excision.
- Sublesional glucocorticoid injections (see above).
- Prognosis uncertain:
  - May spontaneously regress.
  - Response to glucocorticoids variable.
  - Rarely recurs.

Nodular panniculitis/steatitis

Clinical features
- Rare inflammatory condition affecting subcutaneous adipose tissue.
- No age, breed, or sex predilection.
- Cause:
  - Multifactorial: skin infections, immune-mediated conditions (lupus, drug eruption, vasculitis), physicochemical factors (trauma, pressure, cold, foreign body, injection of bulky, oily, or insoluble liquids), systemic disease (pancreatitis), glucocorticoid therapy, nutritional (vitamin E deficiency), enteropathy.
  - Idiopathic.
- Signs:
  - Single or multiple, deep-seated nodules affecting trunk, neck, proximal limbs.

- Variable pain and texture.
- Ulceration and draining tracts may develop.
- Variable systemic signs: anorexia, pyrexia, lethargy, depression.

Diagnosis
- History and clinical signs.
- Stained smears of needle aspirates: neutrophils, macrophages containing lipid droplets, occasional multinucleate histiocytic giant cells, background lipid material.
- Excisional skin biopsies for histopathology with special stains and microbial culture to identify infectious causes and rule out other differentials:
  - Pyogranulomatous, suppurative, necrotising or fibrosing panniculitis; lymphoid nodules often present; ceroid material in lipocytes, macrophages, giant cells, and extracellular; dystrophic mineralisation.
- Differentials: eosinophilic granuloma, infectious granulomata, amyloidosis, neoplasia.

Treatment
- Identify and treat underlying causes.
- Glucocorticoids:
  - Prednisolone 1–2 mg/kg once daily by mouth for 2–3 weeks, then alternate-day dosing and taper according to clinical response.
  - Dexamethasone tablets (Dexacortone, Dechra Veterinary Products, off-label use) 0.1 mg/kg by mouth once daily for 2–3 weeks.
- Prognosis uncertain, dependent upon aetiology:
  - Variable response to glucocorticoids in idiopathic cases.
  - Recurrence may occur, requiring ongoing therapy.

Hamartoma (nevus)

Clinical features
- Benign growths consisting of disorganised overgrowth of mature cells and tissues, usually epidermal in origin, likely due to localised embryonic defect.
- Usually solitary lesions, noted within first 6 months of life, found on head, neck, back, thoracic trunk, rump, or legs.
- Reported in Belgian horses.
- Hyperkeratotic plaques, rubbery in texture, may be pedunculated, linear, or smooth (Figure 5.32).

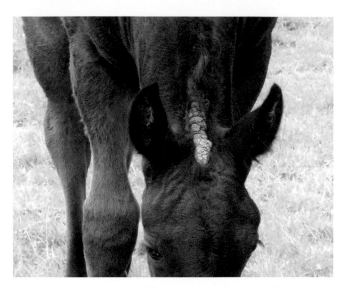

Figure 5.32 Congenital epidermal hamartoma in a Friesian foal. Source: Courtesy of Jacqueline Mortimer.

Diagnosis
- Clinical presentation.
- Histopathology reveals marked hyperkeratosis, papillated epidermal hyperplasia and papillomatosis, without infection or evidence of viral infection; negative for papillomavirus antigen.

Treatment
- Leave and monitor.
- Surgical excision.
- Topical treatment with keratolytic/keratoplastic products such as 50% propylene glycol or retinoid (0.1% tretinoin) cream (off-label use) may give some amelioration of clinical signs.

Calcinosis circumscripta

Clinical features
- Rare.
- Standardbred horses over-represented; young adults 1.5–4 years of age, mostly male horses.
- Cause unknown.

- Signs:
  - Hard, well-circumscribed, subcutaneous nodules 3–20 cm diameter over the lateral stifles, unilateral, bilateral in about one-third of cases, rarely on carpus or tarsus or elsewhere on body. Overlying skin normal.
  - Rarely associated symptoms of local pain or lameness; rarely progressive.

Diagnosis
- Clinical presentation.
- Radiography: localised radio-dense deposits in soft tissues.
- Skin biopsy:
  - Multinodular deposits of mineral separated by fibrosis and granulomatous inflammation.
- Differentials: mineralised eosinophilic granuloma, mineralised mast cell tumours.

Treatment
- Leave alone.
- Surgical excision if symptomatic or for cosmetic reasons; possible complications of septic arthritis, wound dehiscence.

Exuberant granulation tissue (proud flesh)

Clinical features
- Frequent complication of wounds healing by second intention on the distal limbs; overgrowth of granulation tissue above adjacent epithelium.
- Horses at greater risk than ponies.
- Cause:
  - Delayed wound healing associated with chronic inflammation due to bacterial infection, contamination with debris, chemical irritants, inappropriate wound management.
  - Excessive movement, devitalisation of underlying tissues, bone sequestration.
  - Altered cytokine profiles result in increased fibrovascular genesis and reduced myofibroblast differentiation.
- Signs:
  - Proliferation of granulation tissue with no wound contraction, healing, or epithelium production.
  - Tissue is pink to red, firm, and granular.

- Occurs on distal limbs, particularly over areas of high movement – fetlock, flexural surface of tarsus.

Diagnosis
- History of trauma, clinical signs, lesion location.
- Biopsy to rule out other differentials.
- Differentials: fibroblastic sarcoid, habronemiasis, squamous cell carcinoma, infectious granulomata.

Treatment
- Surgical excision of protruding tissue and removal of narrow (2 mm) strip of skin margin to stimulate wound contraction, healing, and re-epithelialisation. Wound dressings – hydrogels, hydrocolloids – to keep surface moist.
- Control infection, pre-operative antibiotics, systemic or regional limb perfusion; local application of glucocorticoid, 1% hydrocortisone ointment every 7 days.
- Support bandages to limit movement and further trauma.
- Skin grafts will accelerate healing and reduce scar formation.
- Prognosis guarded, improved by early grafting; risk of concurrent sarcoid development.
- Prevention:
  - Proper wound management – lavage, debridement, control of infection.
  - Closure of wounds by primary or delayed primary closure where possible.
  - Careful management of large wounds at high risk sites, dressings, pressure bandage, and confine to stable to reduce movement; daily bandage changes initially; additional debridement as needed.
  - Silicone gel dressings once wound defect is filled with healthy granulation tissue bed will reduce likelihood of overgrowth; bandage changes every 2–3 days.

Chronic progressive lymphoedema

Clinical features
- Condition of distal limb of draught horse breeds similar to chronic lymphoedema of humans.
- Reported in Belgian, Clydesdale, Shire, Ardenner, and Gypsy Vanner horses; no sex predisposition; early signs from 2-4 years old, progression of clinical signs throughout life.

- Likely genetically determined; healthy horses of affected breeds have lower levels of the elastin cross-linking amino acid desmosine compared to unaffected breeds.
- Role of chorioptic mange is uncertain as draught breeds are predisposed to both conditions.
- Bacterial infection common, but staphylococcal pyoderma is common in non-pigmented distal limbs and so may co-exist or even predispose to chronic sequelae.
- Cause:
  - Alterations in dermal and lymphatic elastin; interstitial fluid stasis, delayed lymphatic drainage, high anti-elastin antibody levels.
  - Resultant fibrosis, epidermal hyperplasia and hyperkeratosis, increased susceptibility to infection.
- Signs:
  - Early lesions: mild swelling, and scaling of all four distal limbs, hind limbs worse; may not be recognised unless feathered hair is clipped (Figure 5.33).

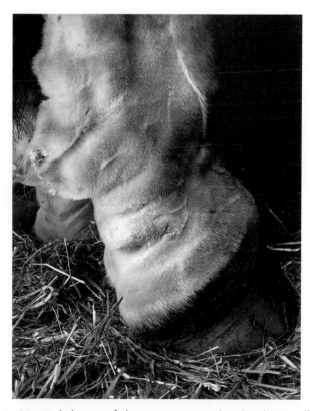

Figure 5.33 Early lesions of chronic progressive lymphoedema. Diffuse swelling of the distal pastern regions of an aged Shire horse, with some surface scaling and coronary band changes.

- Development of skin folds on caudal pasterns, progressing to further swelling, firm thickening of skin due to fibrosis, formation of nodules, ulceration.
- Chronic lesions: nodular thickening encircling distal limb, spreading proximally, marked verrucous hyperkeratosis and scaling (Figure 5.34).
- Secondary bacterial infection in skin folds; often mixed infection including anaerobes.
- Involvement of coronary bands results in abnormal hoof wall growth.
- Pain and lameness.

Diagnosis
- History and clinical findings in draught breed.
- Skin biopsies to confirm.

Treatment
- No curative treatment; palliative treatment to slow progression:
  - Aggressive treatment of bacterial infection; continuing thorough and regular cleansing of skin surface with antiseptic products (see Chapter 3).

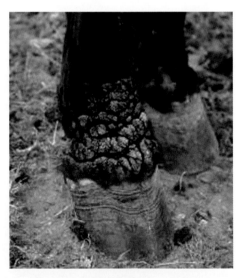

Figure 5.34 Chronic progressive lymphoedema. Multiple fibrotic corrugations and nodules with surface scaling affecting the pastern regions of a Friesian horse that suffered repeated episodes of bacterial infection; involvement of the coronary band region and long-standing nature of condition can be seen by growth irregularities affecting proximal one-half of the hoof wall.

– Control of chorioptic mage if present (see Chapter 2).
– Massage and pressure bandaging to encourage lymphatic drainage.
• Prognosis guarded to poor:
– Euthanasia on humane grounds in severe and chronic cases.
• Prevention: review breeding programmes in light of breed and familial incidence.

Chronic proliferative pododermatitis (canker)

Clinical features
• A rare, chronic, hyperproliferative dermatitis initially affecting caudal part of cleft of frog, progressing to extend to the sole and adjacent hoof walls, affecting one or more feet of any breed of horse, but with a marked prevalence for draught breeds (Figure 5.35).
• Aetiology remains uncertain; spirochaetes and anaerobic bacteria have been identified in cases, but a causal association not established. Consistent detection of bovine papilloma virus (BPV) DNA reported in hoof, skin, and peripheral blood mononuclear cells of affected horses but not controls, but subsequent study showed no statistical difference in detection of BPV DNA between horn tissue from affected animals compared to unaffected.

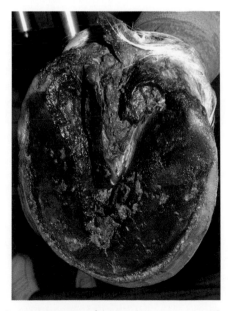

Figure 5.35 Canker. Solar aspect of the hoof showing a proliferative lesion affecting the frog. Source: Courtesy of Richard J. Payne.

- Humidity, unhygienic stabling, and poor hoof care recognised as contributory factors, but disease is not confined to poorly cared-for horses.
- Chronic cases present with foul-smelling, necrotic, and proliferative vegetative lesions of the frog, associated with secondary infection. Lameness may be seen at this stage of disease.

Diagnosis
- Clinical signs.
- Histopathological features consist of dyskeratosis of epithelial cells, with proliferation of the corium and epithelium characterised by hyperplastic, papillomatous acanthosis with parakeratotic hyperkeratosis.
- Differentials: pemphigus foliaceus, coronary band dystrophy, thrush.

Treatment
- Debridement and topical antimicrobial treatment and dressings.
- Regular foot hygiene and farriery care; may need special shoeing.
- Improve stable management.

REFERENCES AND FURTHER READING

BEVA resources for vets Protect ME antimicrobial policy guidance, www. beva.org.uk//Portals/0/Documents/ResourcesForVets/1beva-antimicrobial-policy-template-distributed.pdf.

Combarros, D., Wilhelmi-Vilarrasa, I., Lacroux, C. et al. (2020) Multinodular malignant cutaneous mast cell tumor in a horse with generalized pruritus and reactive fibrosis: A case report. *Journal of Equine Veterinary Science*, 87: 102921. doi: 10.1016/j.jevs.2020.102921.

Elbahi, A., Kipar, A. and Ressel, L. (2018) Histocytic-like atypical mast cell tumours in horses. *Journal of Comparative Pathology*, 162: 14–17.

Greenwood, S., Chow-Lockerbie, B., Epp, T. et al. (2020) Prevalence and Prognostic impact of *Equus caballus* Papillomavirus Type 2 infection in Equine Squamous Cell Carcinomas in Western Canadian Horses. *Veterinary Pathology*, 57 (5): 623–631.

Hollis, A.E. (2019) Radiotherapy for the treatment of periocular tumours in the horse. *Equine Veterinary Education*, 31: 647–652.

Limeira, C.H., Alves, C.J., Azevedo, S.S. et al. (2019) Clinical aspects and diagnosis of leishmaniasis in equids: a systematic review and meta-analysis. *Revista Brasileira de Parasitologia Veterinária*, 28: 574–581.

Littlewood, J.D., Whitwell, K.E., and Day, M.J. (1995) Equine cutaneous lymphoma: A case report. *Veterinary Dermatology*, 6 (2): 105–111. doi:10.1111/j.1365-3164.1995.tb00051.x

Lloyd, D.H. and Page, S.W. (2018) Antimicrobial stewardship in veterinary medicine. *Microbiology Spectrum*, 6 (3). doi: 10.1128/microbiolspec.ARBA-0023-2017.

Luethy, D., Frimberger, A.E., Bedenice, D. et al. (2019) Retrospective evaluation of clinical outcome after chemotherapy for lymphoma in 15 equids (1991–2017). *Journal of Veterinary Internal Medicine*, 33: 953–960.

Mhadhbi, M. and Sassi, A. (2020) Infection of the equine population by *Leishmania* parasites. *Equine Veterinary Journal*, 52: 28–33.

Onen, E.A. (2020) Molecular typing of equine papillomavirus and autovaccination to treat horses with cutaneous papillomatosis. *Australian Veterinary Journal*, 98: 405–410.

Pettersson, C.M., Broström, H., Humblot, P. et al. (2020) Topical treatment of equine sarcoids with imiquimod 5% cream or *Sanguinaria canadensis* and zinc chloride — an open prospective study. *Veterinary Dermatology*, 31: 471-e126.

Pilsworth, R.C. and Knottenbelt, D. (2007) Skin diseases refresher: Urticaria. *Equine Veterinary Education* AE: 151–154.

Raidal, S.L. (2019) Antimicrobial stewardship in equine practice. *Australian Veterinary Journal*, 97: 238–242.

Sullins, K.E. (2020) Melanocytic tumours in horses. *Equine Veterinary Education*, 12: 624–630.

van Brantegem, L., de Cock, H.E., Affolter, V.K. et al. (2007) Antibodies to elastin peptides in sera of Belgian Draught horses with chronic progressive lymphoedema. *Equine Veterinary Journal*, 39: 418–421.

Coat Problems

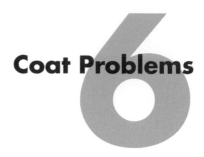

The maintenance of normal coat density is dependent upon the ordered cyclical activity of hair follicles, which, except in areas of hair specialisation, e.g. mane and tail, pass through a growth phase – anagen, a transitional phase – catagen, and a third or resting phase – telogen. Hair growth continues until its pre-ordained length is reached. Shedding of the mature hair is triggered by the growth of a new anagen hair. Hair replacement in horses is mosaic in pattern, predominantly affected by photoperiod, with a prominent shed in the spring in temperate climates. Mane and tail hair, and fetlock hair in cob and heavy breeds, is permanent and not shed in the seasonal pattern of body hair.

ALOPECIA

Definition
- Loss of hair:
    - Total loss of hair affecting a normally hirsute area.
    - A decrease in the number of hairs, or hairs shorter than normal or of reduced diameter: this may be termed hypotrichosis.

Congenital/hereditary conditions
Congenital hypotrichosis

Clinical features
- Rarely reported.

Practical Equine Dermatology, Second Edition. Janet D. Littlewood, David H. Lloyd and J. Mark Craig.
© 2022 John Wiley & Sons Ltd. Published 2022 by John Wiley & Sons Ltd.

- Anecdotally reported in certain lines of Arab horses.
- Reported in a blue roan Percheron:
  - Progressive patchy alopecia of trunk and limbs.
  - Normal teeth and hooves.

Diagnosis
- Clinical presentation.
- Histopathological examination of skin biopsies.

Treatment
- No effective treatment.
- Affected animals should not be used for breeding.

Follicular dysplasia

Clinical features
- Rarely reported.
  - Mane and tail follicular dysplasia seen within a few weeks of age in Appaloosas and animals with curly coat phenotype.
  - Black or white hair follicular dysplasia; short, brittle hair coat in affected colour areas progressing to hypotrichosis and alopecia.

Diagnosis
- Clinical presentation.
- Confirmation by histopathological examination of skin biopsies.
- Differentials: alopecia areata (see below).

Treatment
- No effective treatment.
- Affected animals should not be used for breeding.

Seasonal asynchronous shedding

Clinical features
- Premature loss of telogen hairs in spring before new anagen hairs become visible at the skin surface (Figures 6.1a and b).
- Maybe seen in Thoroughbreds and other fine coated breeds in early spring.
- Patchy alopecia or hypotrichosis over the trunk; underlying skin is normal.

Diagnosis
- Clinical presentation.
- Histopathological examination of skin biopsies not usually necessary.

(a)   (b)

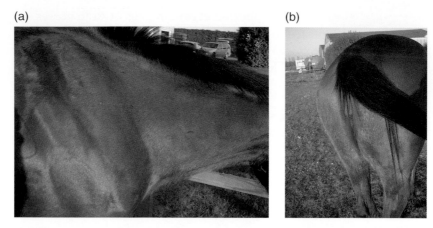

Figure 6.1   a) and **b)** Seasonal asynchronous shedding. Patches of alopecia and hypotrichosis affecting, neck, trunk, and hindquarters of a Thoroughbred mare; the condition recurred every spring. Source: Courtesy of Rob Pilsworth.

- Differentials: malnutrition, early alopecia areata, telogen and anagen effluvium.

Treatment
- None necessary, normal hair coat is seen within days to weeks.

Acquired alopecia

Virtually any inflammatory disease of the skin will precipitate hair loss. Many of these are considered elsewhere. Examples are given below. Many of these conditions cause only temporary alopecia, but ischaemic damage to hair follicles may result in permanent alopecia or hypotrichosis. Permanent cicatricial alopecia may be seen with severe dermal insults that result in loss of follicles due to scarring, e.g. chemical or thermal burn injuries.

- Parasitic infestation: chorioptic mange, pediculosis, larval nematode dermatitis (*Pelodera strongyloides*, *Strongyloides westeri*), onchocerciasis, ticks.
- Infections: dermatophilosis, dermatophytosis, dermatomycosis.
- Immunological reactions: *Culicoides* hypersensitivity, atopic dermatitis, cutaneous lupus erythematosus, eosinophilic enteritis/dermatitis, systemic/localised granulomatous disease, alopecia areata (see below).
- Drug reactions.
- Contact dermatitis (Figure 6.2).
- Neoplasia.

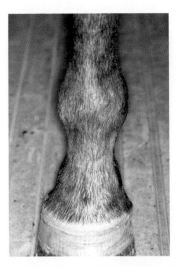

Figure 6.2 Contact irritant dermatitis resulting in diffuse thinning of the haircoat and scaling on the distal limb after application of multiple topical therapies. Note also depigmentation of the proximal hoof wall.

- Toxicoses. heavy metal poisoning, selenium.
- Malnutrition.
- Systemic illness.

Telogen and anagen defluxion (effluvium)

Clinical features

- Synchronised loss of telogen hair may occur due to a disease process or in circumstances of environmental or nutritional stress (e.g. fever, pregnancy, shock, surgery, severe illness). Premature cessation of many anagen hair follicles and synchronisation in telogen results in hair loss within 1–3 months of the insult as the new wave of hair follicle activity begins.
- More severe disease processes and some forms of medication (e.g. chemotherapeutic agents) may precipitate hair loss in the growth phase of the hair follicle cycle – anagen defluxion (Figure 6.3). Hair loss occurs suddenly due to breakage of hair shafts within days of the insult.
- Signs:
  - Regional, multifocal, or generalised alopecia or hypotrichosis.
  - Hair coat easily epilated.
  - Skin surface usually smooth in telogen defluxion, but stubbled hairs can usually be felt with anagen defluxion.

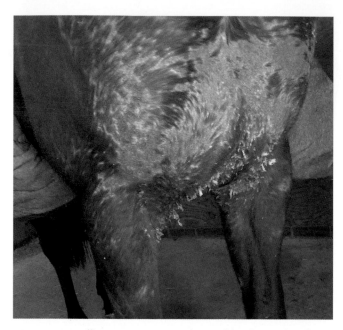

Figure 6.3 Anagen effluvium in a young Thoroughbred. Hair loss began within a week of becoming severely unwell with a postoperative MRSA infection and starting antibiotic treatment; extensive generalised alopecia with easily epilated hair and some exfoliation as hair was shed, but leaving normal underlying epidermis.

Diagnosis

- History and clinical signs.
- Microscopic examination of hairs; either normal telogen hairs present or dysplastic hair shafts with irregular narrowing and deformity of the proximal ends with absence of normal anagen or telogen roots due to fracture.
- Skin biopsy rarely helpful as normal hair follicle activity is usually seen in both conditions, although abnormalities of hair bulbs and dysplastic hair shafts may be present in anagen defluxion.

Treatment

- No specific treatment required; spontaneous resolution occurs when underlying inciting factor(s) is/are eliminated.

Alopecia areata

Clinical features

- An unusual to rare cell-mediated skin disease.
- T-lymphocytes infiltrate around and invade the hair bulb and matrix.

- Signs:
  - Non-scaling, circumscribed areas of alopecia, which may be bilaterally symmetrical, often starting on the face (Figure 6.4), but may become extensive (Figure 6.5). Underlying skin surface is normal.
  - Thinning of mane and tail hair (Figure 6.6).
  - Intermittent periods of remission and recrudescence may occur.
  - Rarely, loss of entire haircoat is seen (alopecia universalis).
  - Possibility of leucotrichia and, or, hoof deformity.

Diagnosis

- History and clinical findings.
- Histopathology of biopsy specimen from the edge of a new lesion to confirm lymphocytic bulbitis.
- Differentials: telogen and anagen effluvium; follicular dysplasia; injection reaction; other drug reaction; occult sarcoid; early localised granulomatous disease; infectious folliculitides (surface changes of scaling and crusting that typically accompany these are absent in alopecia areata).

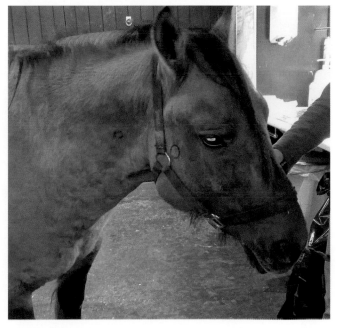

Figure 6.4 Alopecia areata. Facial alopecia and patchy alopecia of the neck and mane.

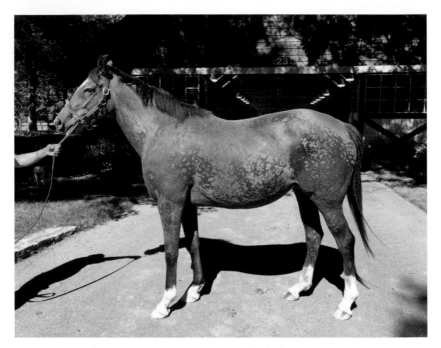

Figure 6.5   Alopecia areata. Extensive generalised alopecia.

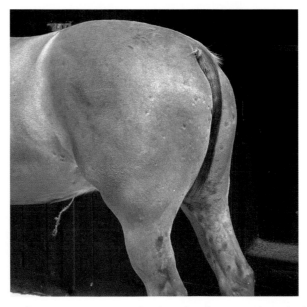

Figure 6.6   Alopecia areata. Generalised patchy alopecia with marked alopecia of the tail.

Treatment
- Immunosuppressive therapy may be considered, but, as the condition is of cosmetic concern only, the potential risks may not justify treatment.
- Corticosteroids are of uncertain efficacy; systemic, topical, or lesional:
  - Prednisolone 1–2 mg/kg by mouth once daily.
  - Topical hydrocortisone aceponate spray (Cortavance, Virbac) applied to lesional areas once daily for up to 1 week then three times weekly (off-label use).
  - Topical triamcinolone spray (Dermanolon, Dechra) used as above (off-label use).
  - Lesional subcutaneous injections of methylprednisolone acetate or triamcinolone (both off-label uses); depot injections carry the greatest risk of side effect of laminitis.
- Topical tacrolimus 0.1% ointment (Protopic, Leo Pharma) applied twice weekly (unlicensed use of human drug) may be beneficial and avoids potential atrophic effects of topical glucocorticoids.
- Minoxidil 2% liquid, lotion, or foam (Rogaine for Women, Johnson & Johnson), applied twice daily may be effective (unlicensed use of non-prescription human drug).

Prognosis
- Treatment may be ineffectual.
- Spontaneous hair regrowth may occur, sometimes with initial, or permanent, leucotrichia.

Toxicoses
Selenosis

Clinical features
- Selenium toxicosis can result from the ingestion of grasses and cereal grains containing excessive selenium due to high soil content of selenium or the presence of selenium-concentrating plants. It has also occurred with wrongly formulated feed additives.
- Occasionally, concentrate feeds may be over-supplemented with selenium. Feed concentrations should not exceed 5 ppm.
- Cutaneous changes are more likely to be seen in chronic toxicity.
- Signs:
  - Whilst a rough, dry haircoat with some skin scaling is seen, the predominant signs are coronary band inflammation, hoof wall changes with variable accompanying lameness, and progressive loss of mane, tail, and fetlock hair (Figures 6.7 and 6.8).
  - Generalised alopecia may develop.

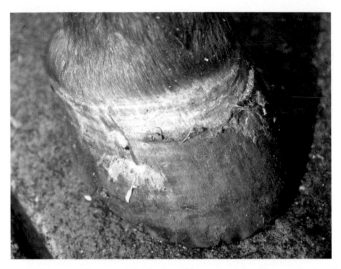

Figure 6.7   Chronic selenosis with abnormal horn growth affecting the hoof wall and shedding of surface layers of keratin. Source: Courtesy of S.C. Shaw.

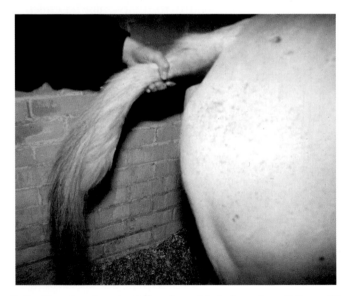

Figure 6.8   Chronic selenosis. Diffuse loss of hair from the tail ('rat tail'). Source: Courtesy of S.C. Shaw.

- Systemic signs may occur and include lethargy, weight loss, and, ultimately, death.

Diagnosis
- History, clinical examination.
- Selenium levels in blood, hoof, and hair:

- Toxic tissue concentrations, typically 1–4 ppm in blood, 11–45 ppm in hair and 8–20 ppm in hoof horn. Selenium may also be found in the urine.
- Differentials: heavy metal toxicity.

Treatment
- There is no specific treatment for chronic selenosis.
- Change diet to reduce intake of selenium.
- Supportive treatments include:
  - Diet high in sulphur-containing amino acids, e.g. methionine supplements.
  - Addition of 5 ppm arsenic to drinking water has been recommended, but is of doubtful efficacy and risks possible arsenic toxicity.
- Recovery is prolonged and euthanasia may be indicated in animals with severe hoof deformities.

Arsenic toxicosis

Clinical features
- Now a rare condition.
- Cutaneous absorption of arsenic causes irritation, drying, and fissuring of the skin.
- Signs:
  - Hair loss, typically over the mane and tail, is seen, although on occasions a hirsute appearance (hypertrichosis) results.
  - Scaling and greasiness, sometimes ulceration.

Diagnosis
- Based on history, clinical signs and renal or hepatic arsenic concentrations >10 ppm.
- Differentials: selenosis, mercury and other toxicoses, pituitary pars intermedia dysfunction (PPID, Cushing's disease), malnutrition.

Treatment
- Removal of source of arsenic.
- D-penicillamine at a dose of 11 mg/kg by mouth daily for 7–10 days (unlicensed treatment).
- Alternative therapies:
  - Sodium thiosulphate, 10–30 g intravenously then 20–60 g by mouth every 6 h for 3–4 days (unlicensed treatment).
  - Dimercaprol 3–5 mg/kg intramuscularly every 6 h for 2 days then twice daily for 8 days (unlicensed treatment).

Mercury toxicosis

Clinical features

- Ingestion of grain treated with organic mercurial substances, such as antifungals, may result in chronic mercury poisoning.
- Topical mercury-containing skin dressings (now rare) may be licked off and, or, absorbed percutaneously.
- Signs:
  - Chronic mercury poisoning results in progressive, generalised alopecia and exfoliation without hoof involvement.
  - Systemic signs include gastroenteritis and weight loss.

Diagnosis

- Mercury is concentrated in the kidneys and chronic poisoning may be confirmed post-mortem by tissue concentration >100 ppm.

Treatment

- Identify and remove source of mercury.
- Sodium thiosulphate and dimercaprol are recommended for treatment (unlicensed treatments); see above for dose rates.

OTHER ABNORMALITIES

Hirsutism refers to the growth of coarse hair in regions that are normally glabrous or covered with vellus hair. Excessive hair due to a prolonged anagen growth phase is more correctly termed hypertrichosis.

Pituitary pars intermedia dysfunction (PPID, equine Cushing's disease)

Clinical features

- Progressive neurodegenerative disorder of horses, ponies, and donkeys due to decreasing production of dopamine by the hypothalamus resulting in loss of inhibitory regulation of the pars intermedia of the pituitary gland, leading to hyperplasia and adenoma formation with excessive production of pituitary hormones including adrenocorticotrophic hormone (ACTH).
- Condition of older equids, rare below 15 years of age and increasing prevalence with age, which is the only risk factor.
- No breed or sex predilection.

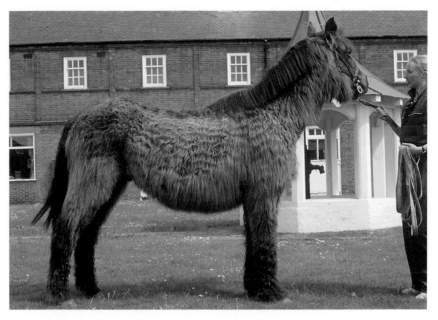

Figure 6.9 Hypertrichosis and pot-bellied appearance in a Connemara pony with PPID.

- Hypertrichosis, with excessively long haircoat due to extended anagen phase and failure to shed, is pathognomonic (Figure 6.9).
- Signs: a range of clinical features may be present:
  - Early PPID.
    - ○ Change in attitude/lethargy.
    - ○ Poor performance.
    - ○ Regional hypertrichosis.
    - ○ Delayed haircoat shedding.
    - ○ Loss of topline muscle.
    - ○ Abnormal sweating (increased or decreased).
    - ○ Infertility.
    - ○ Tendonitis/desmitis.
    - ○ Regional adiposity.
    - ○ Laminitis.
  - Advanced PPID
    - ○ Dull attitude/altered mentation.
    - ○ Exercise intolerance.
    - ○ Generalised hypertrichosis.
    - ○ Loss of seasonal haircoat shedding.
    - ○ Topline muscle atrophy.

- o Rounded/pot-bellied abdomen.
- o Abnormal sweating (increased or decreased).
- o Polyuria, polydipsia.
- o Recurrent infections.
- o Dry eye, recurrent corneal ulcers.
- o Infertility.
- o Increased mammary gland secretions.
- o Tendon and suspensory ligament laxity.
- o Regional adiposity (bulging supraorbital fat).
- o Laminitis, recurrent sole abscesses.
- Concurrent hyperglycaemia (type II diabetes mellitus) may be present; insulin dysregulation is present in approximately one-third of cases, particularly in horses predisposed to equine metabolic syndrome.

Diagnosis
- Clinical appearance in advanced cases may be pathognomonic, but early cases may be difficult to confirm.
- Abnormal laboratory findings that may be present include:
  - Hyperglycaemia
  - Hyperinsulinaemia
  - Hypertriglyceridaemia
  - High faecal egg count
- Measurement of basal ACTH concentration may be diagnostic, but the autumn increase in normal equids requires interpretation in the light of seasonally adjusted cut-off values (see Table 6.1):
  - Blood is collected into EDTA tubes, chill within 3 hours.
  - Sample centrifuged, plasma separated, and transported to the laboratory with ice packs.
- For confirmation when basal values are equivocal the thyrotropin hormone (TRH) stimulation test should be performed. Pharmaceutical grade TRH is not available in the UK; chemical grade TRH can be purchased from https://phoenixpeptide.com/order_information/; the specific product is listed at https://www.phoenixpeptide.com/products/view/Peptides/062-10:
  - Concentrate feed should be withheld for 12 hours prior to testing; can be performed before, but not within 12 hours of undertaking an oral sugar test (OST).
  - Samples taken as above prior to and 10 minutes after intravenous administration of TRH (unlicensed use):
    - o 0.5 mg for animals <250 kg.
    - o 1 mg for animals >250 kg.

Table 6.1 Interpretation of plasma ACTH concentrations (Equine Endocrinology Group updated criteria)

Time of year	PPID unlikely	Interpretive zone	PPID likely
Basal level Non-autumn months*	<15 pg/ml	15-40 pg/ml	>50 pg/ml
Basal level Mid summer and early winter**	<15 pg/ml	15-50 pg/ml	>50 pg/ml
Basal level Late summer***	<20 pg/ml	20-75 pg/ml	>75 pg/ml
Basal level Autumn ****	<30 pg/ml	30-90 pg/ml	>90 pg/ml
Post TRH value Late winter to early summer *****	<100 pg/ml	100-200 pg/ml	>200 pg/ml
Post TRH value Late summer to early winter******	<100 pg/ml	TRH stimulation testing can only be used to identify negative cases in these months due to many false positives	

Key:
* December to June northern hemisphere, June to December southern hemisphere
** July and November northern hemisphere, January and May southern hemisphere
*** August northern hemisphere, February southern hemisphere
**** September and October northern hemisphere, March and April southern hemisphere
***** January to June northern hemisphere, July to December southern hemisphere
****** August to December northern hemisphere, February to June southern hemisphere

Treatment
- Pergolide (Prascend, Boehringer Ingelheim Animal Health), a dopamine receptor agonist, is licensed for the treatment of PPID. Initial dose of 2 μg/kg (0.5 mg for 250 kg pony, 1 mg for 500 kg horse) given once daily by mouth:
  - Some animals show transient inappetence, in which case medication should be discontinued until appetite returns or decrease dose by half for 3–5 days.
  - If no improvement noted within 1–2 months (improved attitude, increased activity, reduced polydipsia/polyuria, improved glucose and insulin dynamics, decreases in basal and post-TRH plasma ACTH) then daily dose can be increased by 1–2 μg/kg with reassessment after further 30 days.
  - Dose may be increased incrementally to a total dose of 6 μg/kg (3 mg/day for 500 kg horse).
- In cases where the response is still suboptimal and endocrine results remain abnormal, addition of cyproheptadine (unlicensed use),

0.25 mg/kg twice daily or 0.5 mg/kg once daily by mouth, may be effective or gradual increase in pergolide dose up to 10 µg/kg daily.
- Clinical signs may improve without endocrine abnormalities returning to normal; regular measurement of blood glucose concentrations and ACTH (non-autumn months) is advised.
- Control of blood glucose in response to pergolide should be assessed before considering other treatments for hyperglycaemia.
- Attention to general health and wellness to include management of secondary infections, monitoring of body condition score, dental care, parasite control, and regular hoof trimming; laminitic animals may require specialist/remedial farriery attention.
- Diet should be adjusted according to body condition scores (BCS):
  - Lean animals with normal insulin status may be fed with senior feeds and pasture grazing.
  - Obese animals (BCS ≥7/9) should receive a low energy diet and an exercise programme.
  - Cases with insulin dysregulation require lower non-structural carbohydrate feeds and limited access to pasture.
- Awareness of welfare status is important; medical management may improve quality of life, but does not necessarily increase longevity. Chronic laminitis, recurrent intractable infections, and poor response to therapy are indications for humane euthanasia.

REFERENCES AND FURTHER READING

Equine Endocrinology Group 2019 Recommendations on diagnosis and management for pituitary pars intermedia dysfunction (PPID). https://sites.tufts.edu/equineendogroup/files/2019/12/2019-PPID_EEGbooklet.pdf

Equine Endocrinology Group 2020 Recommendations on diagnosis and management for equine metabolic syndrome (EMS) including assessment of insulin status. https://sites.tufts.edu/equineendogroup/files/2020/09/200592_EMS_Recommendations_Bro-FINAL.pdf

Pigmentary Disorders

GENETICS OF SKIN AND COAT COLOUR

Pigmented hair

Melanin is produced in melanocytes in the basal layer of the epithelium and hair bulb and transferred to epidermal cells or cells of the hair matrix, respectively. Pigmentation in hair shafts may be influenced by different or additional genes from those affecting the skin pigment.

The basic coat colours in the horse are influenced by the interaction between two genes: Melanocortin 1 Receptor (*MC1R*), also known as the extension or black/red factor locus, and Agouti Signalling Protein (*ASIP*).

- *MC1R* controls production of black or red pigment; three alleles recognised:
  - *E* is dominant to *e* and e^a, resulting in production of black hairs.
  - Homozygous recessive individuals (*e/e* or e^a/e^a) produce only red hairs.
- *ASIP* controls the distribution of black hair.
  - Dominant allele *A* restricts black pigment to the points (mane, tail, lower limbs, ear margins).
  - Recessive form (*a*) distributes black pigment uniformly over the body.
- Basic coat colours are chestnut (*e/e* or e^a/e^a), bay (*E* and *A*), and black (*E* and *a/a*).
- Variability in shades of pigmentation is influenced by many genes, not yet fully elucidated.

Practical Equine Dermatology, Second Edition. Janet D. Littlewood, David H. Lloyd and J. Mark Craig.
© 2022 John Wiley & Sons Ltd. Published 2022 by John Wiley & Sons Ltd.

- Several dilution genes affect the amount of pigment produced or transferred to hair follicle cells. Six phenotypes have been characterised including:
  - Cream (*Cr*), which is dominant:
    - A single copy (*N/Cr*) produces yellow colour – palomino on a chestnut background or buckskin (with black points) on a bay background.
    - Two copies (*Cr /Cr*) produce pale cream colour – cremellos on a chestnut background, perlinos on a bay background, and smoky creams on a black background with pink skin.
  - Dun (*D*) is dominant and dilutes the coat colour of the trunk, leaving points unaffected, and includes primitive markings of a dorsal stripe.
    - Horses with *nd1* without *D* are not dun dilute, but may have primitive markings.
    - Animals with *nd2/nd2* are not dun dilute and do not have primitive markings.

White hair

There are several genes responsible for white haircoat patterns. White hair patterns can be divided into:

- Distributed or intermixed.
  - Includes roan and grey, which are both dominant mutations:
    - Roans have white hairs distributed throughout the coat, although the face may be fully pigmented. The pattern is present from birth or shortly after.
    - Grey horses progressively lose hair pigment with age whilst skin remains pigmented; they are at risk of developing melanoma.
- Patch patterns, also caused by dominant mutations including:
  - Dominant White mutation of the Kit gene (*W*), with various variant alleles, which confers inability to form pigment, gives white hair and pink skin; includes piebald and skewbald patterns seen in the UK. Can be additionally modified by the presence of additional genes.
  - Overo gene (*O*) present in frame overo, tovero, and tobiano patterns.
  - Various genes control other spotted patterns (leopard complex gene of the Appaloosa, sabino, splashed white).

Genetic testing

Tests for various genes involved in equine hair coat colour are available.

- Veterinary Genetics Laboratory, University of California Davis https://vgl.ucdavis.edu/resources/horse-coat-color

- Animal Genetics UK https://www.animalgenetics.eu/Equine/Coat_Colour/Colour_Index.asp
- Laboklin UK https://www.laboklin.co.uk/laboklin/GeneticDiseases.jsp

HYPOPIGMENTATION DISORDERS

Definitions:
- Leucoderma: absence of skin pigment.
- Leucotrichia: absence of hair pigment.

Hereditary and congenital disorders
Lethal white foal disease

Clinical features
- Homozygosity for the frame overo allele (*O/O*) confers a lethal phenotype.
- Reported in American Paint horses, Pintos, and Quarter horses.
- Foals are white with accompanying gastrointestinal tract abnormalities.
- Gut defects include ileocolonic aganglionosis, myenteric aganglionosis, intestinal aganglionosis.
- Affected foals are born apparently normal but develop colic after a variable period due to gut stasis and inability to pass faeces. Affected gut is contracted and functional obstruction is present.
- Death occurs in 1–5 days.

Diagnosis
- Clinical presentation.
- Differentiate from failure to pass meconium and distal intestinal atresia, which can occur in foals of any colour.
- Confirm by genetic testing.

Treatment
- No effective treatment; euthanasia is indicated.
- Parents should be removed from breeding programmes or only bred if not carrying the frame overo allele.

Lavender foal syndrome (LFS; coat colour dilution lethal, CCDL)

Clinical features
- Rare hereditary congenital condition of Arab foals with Egyptian bloodlines.

- Foals are born with diluted haircoat colour varying from silver to lavender, pale slate grey, or pale chestnut (pink).
- Various neurological abnormalities are present including inability to assume sternal recumbency, opisthotonus, paddling, extensor rigidity, seizures, and blindness.

Diagnosis
- Clinical presentation of severe neurological defects with characteristic coat colour.
- Confirmation by DNA test for mutation in the myosin Va gene, which affects the function of melanocytes and neurons.
- Differential diagnoses: head trauma, neonatal maladjustment syndrome.

Treatment
- No effective treatment; euthanasia is indicated.
- Parents should be removed from breeding programmes or only bred if not carrying the LFS gene.

Acquired pigmentary disorders

Non-pigmented skin has an increased susceptibility to damage as a result of exposure to ultraviolet radiation. These conditions are covered in Chapter 3 (Crusting and scaling disorders).

Most cases of acquired leucoderma and leucotrichia are post-inflammatory in nature. The inflammatory insult may arise as a result of a number of initiating factors with subsequent damage to melanocytes in the epidermis and, or, hair follicle, some examples of which follow.

Physical and chemical causes

- Cold branding, cryosurgery, burns.
- Trauma:
  - Wounds from ill-fitting harness and tack, plaster casts, bandages (Figure 7.1) rope burns, deep skin wounds.
- Chemical agents:
  - Blisters, rubber toxicity, primary irritant contact dermatitis (Figure 7.2).

Infectious causes
Parasitic

- Trypanosomiasis – *Trypanosoma equiperdum* infection (dourine): genital infection of males and females, ulceration of genitalia with depigmentation, urticarial wheals on the neck, shoulders, and back,

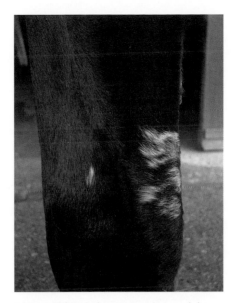

Figure 7.1 Leucotrichia and focal alopecia on the caudal carpus secondary to damage due to bandage injury.

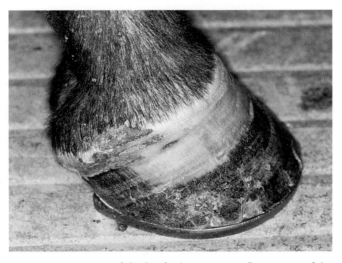

Figure 7.2 Depigmentation of the hoof subsequent to inflammation of the coronary band due to contact irritant reaction after multiple topical therapies applied to the distal limb.

occurring in most of Asia, northern and southern Africa, Russia, parts of the Middle East, South America, and Southeastern Europe.
- Onchocerciasis: ventral midline dermatitis.
- Parafilariasis: *Parafilaria multipapillosa* infestation, seasonal cutaneous larval migration.

Bacterial and fungal

- Deep infections leading to ulceration. Healing accompanied by permanent depigmentation.

Viral

- Aural plaques – papovavirus infection. *Simulium* flies act as vectors.
- Coital exanthema – EHV-3 infection: papular, vesicular, and pustular lesions on the genitals of mare and stallion. Oral, nostril, and lip lesions are occasionally seen. Healed lesions show permanent depigmentation.

Immune-mediated

- *Culicoides* hypersensitivity (sweet itch) (Figure 7.3).
- Cutaneous lupus erythematosus (see Chapter 3).
- Erythema multiforme (see Chapter 3).

Vitiligo

Clinical features
- Uncommon condition reported in several breeds of horses, including Arabs (Arabian fading syndrome, pinky syndrome), Belgian Tervuerens, Gelderlanders, and Thoroughbreds.

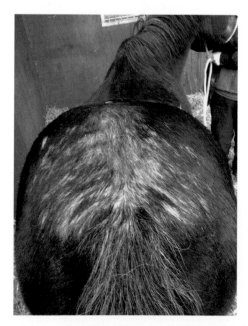

Figure 7.3   Leucotrichia on the caudo-dorsal rump of a pony with a long history of *Culicoides* hypersensitivity (sweet itch).

- Wide age range, but most common in young adult animals; possible predisposition for females.
- Antibodies against melanocyte surface antigens have been demonstrated and cell-mediated mechanisms also involved.
- Other mechanisms also proposed, including a neural theory and nutrient deficiencies, but with little supportive evidence.
- Signs:
  - Annular areas of macular depigmentation usually involving head, often with mucocutaneous distribution.
  - May also affect other areas of the body, including genital and perineal mucocutaneous regions (Figures 7.4 a and b); hooves may also be affected.
  - Affected skin otherwise normal.

Diagnosis
- Clinical findings.
- Skin biopsies early in disease may show lymphocytic inflammation involving upper dermis and basal epidermis with apoptosis of melanocytes; later in the course of disease may only see absence of melanocytes and melanin in the epidermis.

Treatment
- Degree of depigmentation may wax and wane, and some animals will spontaneously completely re-pigment.
- Anecdotal reports of benefits from increased dietary vitamin A and copper are difficult to interpret because of the natural waxing and waning and spontaneous remission that may occur.

(a) (b)

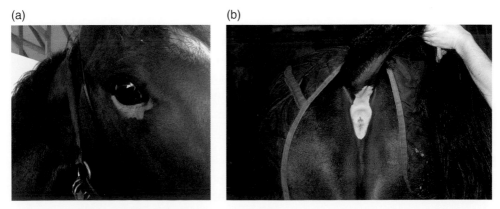

Figure 7.4 Vitiligo. Periocular depigmentation (a) and perianal depigmentation (b). The horse also had patchy leucoderma of the muzzle and penis.

Keratinisation disorders

Linear keratosis – areas of crusting, hair loss, and subsequent depigmentation (see Chapter 3).

Conditions of uncertain aetiology
Spotted leucotrichia

Clinical features
• Uncommon, poorly characterised disorder reported in many breeds, particularly Arab horses, Thoroughbreds, and Shire horses.
• Annular spots of white hair 1–3 cm diameter affecting dorso-lateral trunk.
• No associated skin lesions, leucoderma not usually present.
• May be a form of vitiligo.

Diagnosis
• Clinical findings.
• Histopathology not well-defined.

Treatment
• No known effective treatment.

Reticulated leucotrichia

Clinical features
• Uncommon condition of unknown cause, but breed predispositions suggest a genetic role.
• Seen in Quarter horses, Thoroughbreds, Standardbreds, and occasionally other breeds.
• Occurs in young horses, no sex predisposition.
• May be an unusual form of erythema multiforme associated with herpesvirus infection and vaccination.
• Signs:
  – Linear crusts in a cross-hatched pattern over the dorsal trunk from withers to tail base; usually asymptomatic, sometimes painful.
  – Shedding of crusts leaves temporary alopecia followed by permanent leucotrichia.

Diagnosis
• History and clinical findings.
• Skin biopsies for histopathological examination taken early in disease may reveal interface dermatitis.

Treatment

- No known effective treatment.

Hyperaesthetic leucotrichia

Clinical features

- Rare condition of unknown aetiology.
- May be a form of erythema multiforme; has been associated with herpesvirus infection and vaccination.
- No breed, age, or sex predisposition.
- Signs:
  - Single or multiple raised crusts on dorsal midline accompanied by extreme pain.
  - Crusts and pain resolve over 1–3 months leaving permanent leucotrichia.

Diagnosis

- Clinical presentation.
- Histopathology of skin biopsies early in disease may show features of erythema multiforme.

Treatment

- No effective treatment reported.
- The condition may recur in some animals.

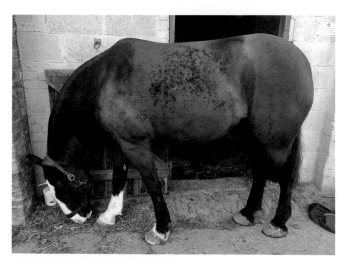

Figure 7.5 Melanotrichia. Tufts of hyperpigmented hairs at sites of earlier inflamed urticarial lesions and resolved secondary folliculitis in an atopic horse. Source: Courtesy of Ms. K. Clarke.

HYPERPIGMENTATION

Melanotrichia

Small areas of dark hairs may occur at sites of inflammatory reactions (Figure 7.5).

REFERENCES AND FURTHER READING

Tham, H.L., Linder, K.E., and Olivry, T. (2019) Autoimmune diseases affecting skin melanocytes in dogs, cats and horses: Vitiligo and the uveo-dermatological syndrome: A comprehensive review. *BMC Veterinary Research*, 15: 251.

Veterinary Genetics Laboratory, University of California Davis.https://vgl.ucdavis.edu/resources/horse-coat-color

Animal Genetics, UK. https://www.animalgenetics.eu/Equine/Coat_Colour/Colour_Index.asp

Therapy in Equine Dermatology

AVAILABILITY OF VETERINARY MEDICINES FOR EQUINE PATIENTS

Background

- The horse is classified in the European Union (EU) as a minor food-producing species; although the UK is no longer in the EU, it is likely that the UK will continue to adhere to EU medicines legislation regarding food-producing animals.
- All horses, apart from semi-wild ponies, must have a passport, in which they can be declared as either intended for human consumption (food-producing) or not intended for human consumption (non-food-producing).
- Whether or not a horse is declared as intended for human consumption determines what medicines can be administered to the animal and what records must be kept.

Prescribing for horses

- In the UK, horses must be treated with veterinary medicines that have a UK marketing authorisation for use in the horse for the condition being treated as the first choice.
- If there is no suitable authorised product available, then veterinary surgeons may prescribe for animals under their care an alternative medicine under the prescribing cascade; the second choice would be a drug licensed for another condition in the horse, or a drug licensed

Practical Equine Dermatology, Second Edition. Janet D. Littlewood, David H. Lloyd and J. Mark Craig.
© 2022 John Wiley & Sons Ltd. Published 2022 by John Wiley & Sons Ltd.

for the condition in a different animal; if no such alternative exists, then a human drug may be prescribed.

- If a medicinal product is to be used in a food-producing animal, then it must have a maximum residue limit (MRL), in addition to a market authorisation (product licence).
- Permitted medications are listed in table 1 of Commission Regulation 37/2010. The ability to use these medicines is usually contained in the SPC (data sheet) insert or via the VMD Product Information Database.
- In addition, there are drugs legally permitted for use in food-producing horses that are included in an essential substance list (Commission Regulation 122/2013). These can only be used with a 6-month withdrawal period.
- Any horse receiving medication that is not included in these lists must be permanently excluded from the food chain and the declaration in the passport signed by the horse owner, its keeper, or the vet.
- Veterinarians, pharmacists, and other suitably qualified persons, when prescribing for horses, must have sight of the passport (unless recently viewed), and be satisfied that the passport relates to the animal to be treated. If the declaration concerning its status as a food-producing animal is not signed, then the animal must be considered to be intended for human consumption. For food-producing animals, the meat withdrawal periods in the SPC (data sheet) must be followed and recorded, although not necessarily in the passport. Drugs listed in table 1 of Regulation EU 37/2101 that are prescribed under the cascade must be recorded in the passport, with a suitable withdrawal period. Details of products with active substances prescribed from the essential list under the cascade must be recorded in the passport, with the date of last administration and owners advised of the statutory 6-month withdrawal period.

REFERENCES AND FURTHER READING

Horse medicines and record-keeping requirements. Guidance produced by the Veterinary Medicines Directorate; originally published 1 June 2015, most recently updated 5 September 2018. https://www.gov.uk/guidance/horse-medicines-and-recording-keeping-requirements

The cascade: prescribing unauthorised medicines. Guidance produced by the Veterinary Medicines Directorate; originally published 1 June

2015, most recently updated 13 January 2021. https://www.gov.uk/guidance/the-cascade-prescribing-unauthorised-medicines

Medicines legislation and passports. Guidance produced by the British Equine Veterinary Association. https://www.beva.org.uk/Guidance-and-Resources/Medicines/Medicines-legislation-and-passports

Index

Note: Page numbers in *italics* indicate figures; those followed by t indicate tables.

Practical Equine Dermatology, Second Edition. Janet D. Littlewood, David H. Lloyd and J. Mark Craig.
© 2022 John Wiley & Sons Ltd. Published 2022 by John Wiley & Sons Ltd.